Women's
OPTIMAL PELVIC HEALTH
with Merciér Therapy

Women's
OPTIMAL PELVIC HEALTH
with Merciér Therapy

Jennifer Merciér, MS, PhD

ISBN: 978-1-60594-619-1

First Printing, 2010; Second Printing, 2011

Quotations on pages 5, 7, 37, 41, 49, 57, and 63 from www.thinkexist.com.

Quotations on pages 11, 15, 23, 29, 53, 59, 71, 75, and 87 from www.quotegarden.com.

Quotations on pages 33, 45, and 67 from www.quotationspage.com.

Quotation on page 79 from *What the River Knows* by Wayne Fields. © 1990, University of Chicago Press, Chicago, p. 66.

Illustrations on pages 27 and 28 from www.healthyuterus.com.

Additional Praise for This Book

"Dr. Jenny is the reason I'm pregnant today. With three things against me: a past c-section, thyroid issues and fertility issues I was pretty sure we were going to be a one child family. Much to mine and my husband's surprise after a few Merciér Therapy treatments and herbal and homeopathic supplements we were pregnant! We cannot thank Dr. Jenny enough for all of her help and support."

—Sara Pomaro
Yoga Instructor, Geneva, Illinois

"There is very little out there on female pelvic and fertility problems that is both knowledgeable and user-friendly; this book successfully straddles both. For the many women and couples out there seeking to find their way in the morass of medical specialties, this book offers a lit path that will eliminate suffering and anguish."

—Tom Myers
Author of *Anatomy Trains*, Elsevier 2001, 2009

"After two miserable c-section experiences, my husband and I decided to pursue having a VBAx2C for the birth our third child. This is no easy task because most medical professionals refuse to attend VBACs at all. We were so blessed to come in contact with a midwife who was willing to attend our birth. Having a baby at home was the most empowering event of my life. There were a few key pieces to our homebirth success. One of which was Merciér Therapy. Dr. Jenny spent time working on my abdomen during my pregnancy to decrease round ligament pain and create a healthier environment for my growing baby by dealing with the adhesions around my section scar. Going to Dr. Jenny helped my physical state and greatly helped me prepare for our successful VBA2C!"

—Amanda Transparenti
Mother of three lovely children

"Merciér Therapy is unique in its direct and comprehensive approach to women's health care. As a chiropractor Merciér Therapy has changed my practice by helping me in the evaluation and treatment of difficult cases of pelvic, hip and low back pain in women. Merciér Therapy is a must for medical professionals that care for women."

—Dr. Amanda Herzer, Chiropractic Physician
Interchange Wellness Center, Chicago, Illinois

"I applaud you in getting this information out there... it will help so many women!"

—Karen Drucker
Inspirational Singer and Songwriter

"Dr. Merciér's book is an insightful and invaluable resource for all women. She weaves her personal struggles with infertility and clinical expertise into this unique book. With the creation of her amazing and clinically proven method, Merciér Therapy, she has helped countless patients to take control of their health and infertility issues. She enables them to see these life changing ramifications in the eyes of their newborn children every day. Spend just a few moments with this practitioner and you will quickly realize why I am honored to call her my colleague and friend. The world is blessed with a health care provider of her caliber, providing beneficial services to women and humanity in general."

—Skip Hart, MS, OMD
Diplomate Naturopathic Medicine, Author and Health Advocate

"I was pleased to read Dr. Merciér's book. I have a great appreciation for the dedication she has to her patients, the comprehensive approach to the emotional and physical aspects of chronic pelvic pain and infertility, and the concepts, thought and creativity she puts into her work. It's clear, she has helped a lot of women, which is what this work is all about."

—Tori Hudson, ND
Medical Director of A Woman's Time
Clinical Professor NCNM, Bastyr U, and SCNM
Author of *Women's Encyclopedia of Natural Medicine*

"*The management of the infertile couple needs to be done in an integrated holistic approach. Getting fit for fertility by addressing all aspects of the couple is essential not only to improve natural conception but also to improve any form of assisted conception that may be required. Jennifer's book is a very welcome addition to the library on infertility. It demonstrates how a holistic approach can occur in practice with the need for excellent communication between different practitioners.*"

—Michael Dooley, MD
Gynecologist and Reproductive Endocrinologist
Author of *Fit For Fertility*
Fellow of the Royal College of Obstetricians and Gynaecologists
Poundbury Fertility Clinic, London

"*In this outstanding work, Dr. Jennifer Merciér explains the female biomechanics in a clear and practical way suitable for clinical application and patient comprehension. I recommend this book to all practitioners seeking to provide more complete care for their perinatal clients.*"

—Jeanne Ohm, DC
Perinatal Practitioner
Executive Director of the International Chiropractic Pediatric Association

Patients: Please note that the information contained in this book is not intended to replace the knowledge and care of a licensed medical practitioner.

Practitioners: Connect with forward-thinking professionals who keep up with current research and theories that support holism. Educate patients to save money by using foods instead of multiple supplements to be their medicine. Know that patients are seeking knowledge to support their wellness. Ultimately, help women understand how to discern the healthiest choices.

Incidents presented in this book are actual experiences. Some names have been changed to protect identities.

*This book is dedicated to my beloved and patient husband, Brian.
I love you.*

*Over the past eleven years in practice I have seen unique situations.
My passion lies with women who have had difficulty conceiving and
who suffer from pelvic pain. My thanks to all the women who have
entrusted me with their holistic fertility care.*

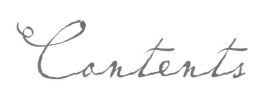

Contents

Introduction

In eighth grade my period began. Nothing eventful ever occurred with my cycles until I was twenty-one. Remembering that time, what comes to mind is agony. My menstrual cycles had taken a turn in an unfamiliar direction. A gynecologist suspected that I was showing symptoms of endometriosis. At that point the remedy for my pain was oral contraceptive pills. The pills did relieve the discomfort for a short while, but another concern surfaced: severe headaches. Typically they would surface a couple days prior to the start of my menstrual cycle and last for an excruciating twenty-four hours. Finally I decided to stop taking the pill and had to contend with pelvic pain again.

At age twenty-three I had my first laparoscopy to determine if endometriosis was growing within my pelvis. Sure enough, I had stage two endometriosis.

As I got further along in my graduate academics, the endometriosis became worse, and another laparoscopy cleaned up the disease. The adhesions and implants, I was told, had grown very aggressive; my endometriosis was now classified as stage three.

Well established in my practice at age thirty-five, I had my third and final laparoscopy. The endometriosis was then a super aggressive stage four. An abundance of scar tissue covered the ovaries and the uterus and surrounding structures. My goal was to get pregnant, and I knew that I needed an expert surgeon to operate. My surgeon was one of the best in the U.S. I appreciated his careful technique and trusted him to preserve my fertility. Sitting in the reproductive endocrinologist's office and listening to him recap my surgery was daunting. He believed he cleared out everything as well as he could without upsetting the delicate ovarian surface. Once the ovaries have been operated on, a thin covering of scar tissue likely forms. This fibrous scar tissue is tough and can create a barrier that would inhibit ovulation. A follicle can grow on the ovary but may not be able to rupture through that tough scar tissue into the fallopian tube.

Since I had undergone two prior surgeries, the ovarian surface had sustained some damage. My expert surgeon recommended that Brian and I go directly to in vitro fertilization. I asked what he thought might be realistic as far as trying on our own. How much time should we give ourselves? What could we expect if we did nothing? Here I was, the holistic fertility expert, in the same boat as many of my clients. We had less than 20 percent chance of conceiving on our own with no help, my surgeon said. At best we should use a drug to stimulate my ovarian egg production, trigger my ovulation with HCG, and then do intrauterine inseminations.

Not wanting to use drugs or procedures to help us conceive, we believed IVF was not an option. So we compromised with the doctor. Brian and I felt most at ease with HCG trigger and intrauterine insemination.

Three cycles later I was not pregnant. I decided that I wanted no more medical intervention. Something about the medical care did not sit well with me. It was not that we were not in good hands; it just felt a bit too manipulated for my liking. So with 20 percent as our number, Brian and I went on our way.

I relaxed and continued to eat healthful, organic foods, take my MultiGreens vitamin, use natural progesterone during my luteal phase, drink plenty of water, cut down on my caffeine intake, and use my pelvic therapy technique on myself.

Despite my clockwork periods every twenty-eight days, I kept wondering why I was approaching the thirty-second cycle day and thinking that my breasts were tender. On the way home from my office I picked up the most efficient pregnancy test. I did not want to have to interpret the color of a testing line or have to ask six people to determine the color. The best test for me was the one that said "pregnant" or "not pregnant." While waiting for the hourglass on the testing window to stop spinning, I washed my hands and came back to my result—"pregnant." I was in shock and elated. Voila! At age thirty-five with stage four endometriosis and after three laparoscopies, I was pregnant.

My journey taught me to trust myself and helped me understand the power of the mind, heart, and womb connection.

Part 1

A Conscious Conception

~1~ *Building a Solid Foundation*

*"What lies behind us and what lies before us are
tiny matters compared to what lies within us."*

—Ralph Waldo Emerson

Over my years of practice, so many encouraging experiences
have inspired me to write. Hearing of a positive pregnancy
test is one of the greatest. Today that very thing occurred,
and another happy, pregnant woman is in this beautiful world of ours.
Her story is one of trust and patience. I have a bias toward this way of
thinking. It is a choice to wait and trust that your body knows what
to do with the help of a gentle, holistic nudge. Therein lies a quiet
knowledge of what is possible with a bit of help and understanding.

Start with your heart. Do any unresolved emotional issues need to be addressed prior to becoming pregnant? Are you working too much? How is your diet? Is your relationship solid? Are you ready to make big changes and commit to a regimen that helps naturally enhance your chances of conception?

State of mind is everything and can dictate the energy surrounding a normal menstrual cycle and conception.

If you are reading this book, you have chosen to take a proactive step of taking your fertility into your own hands and are on your way toward building a solid foundation. Bravo to you!

~2~ Educating Yourself

"There's only one corner of the universe you can
be certain of improving, and that's your own self."

—Aldous Leonard Huxley

Awake: completely conscious, vigilant, watchful. Ask yourself if you are awake. Certainly if you are not sleeping, you are awake, right? Literally speaking, yes, you are awake. But are you really? Are you on auto pilot, just coasting through your day? Has your routine become stagnant yet tolerable enough that you just do it? Perception and awareness are going to bring you close to yourself so you can better understand your needs.

Utilize the resources that are within your reach. But how do you know if those resources are good? My best advice is to acknowledge the creator or author's background, training, and experience. If all of those fit your ideals, then go with it. Talking with other women about their paths can also be helpful in guiding you toward a conscious conception.

Your fertility deserves your full attention. Walking into a fertility clinic blindly can be to your detriment; know the questions to ask your care provider. If a doctor suggests that you undergo a specific test, will you be fully prepared? Many times when I take a woman's history, she is not clear about what went on at her RE appointment.

Lab values and ultrasound reports belong to you, so you should have copies of each and every test report. This information is valuable for me to see. It tells me if your egg reserves are acceptable and if your tubes are patent. Consider these important details with great care.

Knowing the normal signs in the menstrual cycle is crucial for conception to occur. My practice sees about thirty couples a year who inquire about their fertility status. It seems that 60 percent of women are not really in touch with the hormonal trends and fertility signs during their menstrual cycle. On the other hand, the remaining 40 percent keep meticulous journals in which they log each cycle. A normal menstrual cycle lasts twenty-eight to thirty days, beginning with the first day of a period. Ovulation, when the egg is released from the ovary, typically occurs halfway through the cycle. Once released, the egg is fertile up to two days. If the egg is not fertilized, the lining of the uterus disintegrates, resulting in the next menstrual period. Signs of fertility are a surge in luteinizing hormone (LH), temperature rise due to an increase in progesterone, and increased cervical mucus.

Oh, and by the way, do you ovulate?

Signs of an anovulatory cycle, meaning you are not ovulating:

- Heavy bleeding during periods
- Infrequent or light periods
- Absent periods
- Reduced or absent PMS symptoms
- Irregular basal body temperature

Knowledge is indeed power. After all, to bring forth all the information needed in making a truly informed decision helps us understand ourselves even more.

~3~ *Choosing a Care Provider*

"Becoming pregnant is not something that happens because of concentrated effort, denial, or sufferance. It is a natural, unfolding process that stems from a relaxed and positive attitude and a body that is in the correct state of equilibrium."

—Jennifer Merciér

Many times we want for something so strongly that it clouds our vision and natural ability to think things through. The order in which life is created is an intricate process. We cannot give up this precious process to a stranger. We do not need to be rescued from ourselves. Most times we just need quality guidance from a trusted care provider.

Seek care from someone who shares your vision of wellness. Throughout the years I have worked with many medical professionals who are unhealthy people. They overeat, overdrink, smoke, and rarely get enough movement to support a healthy body. I cannot help but wonder why a person who is struggling with pain would seek out care from another person who is unhealthy. Have you ever visited a medical professional only to notice that the person was clearly stressed, did not make eye contact with you, and probably was not even listening? The doctor may have gotten out a prescription pad and prescribed a pain medicine and perhaps ordered a test to help with a diagnosis. It is obvious that the care provider was disconnected due to his own fatigue and stress. My point is this: choose carefully when employing a care provider. Fantastic medical professionals are out there. When you are on your search, be prepared to discern who will best take care of you.

Next, when choosing a care provider for fertility assistance, prenatal care, or a gynecological issue, be certain that you are comfortable with that professional. Remember, the professional you have chosen is your employee. If he or she does not make you feel like all of your questions have been answered or brushes you off due to busyness, then fire that person. Find someone you connect with.

Unfortunately I hear from many clients that they are unhappy with medical care they are receiving. I ask them to explain in detail their experience. Once the whole story has been laid out, I proceed with the pertinent questions: Is your provider available for you to ask questions? Does your provider accept you as an integral part of your treatment? Is your provider able to clearly outline your financial obligations? These questions are the top three in my opinion.

Once you have chosen a provider, make sure you are being taken seriously and respected for your choices by revisiting the reason you are seeking help in the first place. Don't lose yourself in the process of conceiving. If you are lost, then where will your baby grow and thrive? Moms and babies are connected. Baby is a unit of mom and feels what mom feels.

~4~ Soft Tissue Massage

"If you surrender to the wind, you can ride it."

—Toni Morrison

In the U.S. infertility is defined as the inability to conceive after twelve months of unprotected sexual intercourse. But internationally that period is longer, generally twenty-four months. It is clear that here in the U.S. we like to rush and make everything convenient for our own agendas. Conception is not a process we can rush. Important preparatory work needs to be done first—most of all, proper balance within the organs of the pelvis. There is a good chance that the uterus may be malpositioned and would greatly benefit from soft tissue massage. Herbs, vitamins, supportive natural hormones, and education are components as well.

Let's talk about soft tissue work and the importance of creating a healthy space. It is estimated that 40 percent of women are affected with mechanical infertility, meaning the actual reproductive organs are not functioning properly. Pelvic adhesions are considered among the primary causes (more than 50 percent) of mechanical infertility. Formed as a natural response to tissue damage caused by surgery, infection, inflammation, or trauma, they are a by-product of the healing process and remain long after the original wound has healed. Adhesions may be on an organ or muscle, perhaps on its surface, or attached to neighboring structures. Wherever they are, they disfigure and distort the reproductive organs and cause a decrease in function.

Pelvic adhesions not only result from surgery but can also be related to endometriosis, pelvic inflammatory disease, polyps, bowel obstruction, polycystic ovary syndrome, and many other conditions. These adhesions may limit the ability to conceive, even when in vitro fertilization or assisted reproductive technologies are used.

Many types of fertility treatments bypass the core problem of poor reproductive organ function. How about using a gentle, corrective massage therapy to create more blood flow and mobility of the uterus, ovaries, and tubes? Does this not make a great deal of sense? Go to the source of the challenge and help fix it, gently and effectively.

Merciér Therapy—site-specific, manual soft tissue therapy—has to occur on a consistent basis to achieve maximum results. Consider someone who has injured her shoulder. Physical therapy would be prescribed. The therapy would be done not just once or twice. For healing to occur, to see change in the joint and muscles, therapy would need to be done two or three times per week for eight weeks. Likewise, I recommend that women do twelve sessions of therapy over a one-month period to achieve the best results. And Merciér Therapy has produced excellent results, facilitating fertility in women with a wide range of adhesion-related infertility and reproductive organ dysfunction. It also improves soft tissue mobility and elasticity and breaks down adhesions that cause pain and dysfunction. A bonus is that the pelvic work is noninvasive and will not disrupt women's medical protocol for IVF or IUI.

A study published in a peer-reviewed journal showed a 71 percent natural pregnancy rate for patients diagnosed with female infertility after they received manual soft tissue therapy. This therapy also assists in gynecological care prior to IVF or IUI treatments, making the procedures more effective.[1]

Pelvic therapy is also beneficial during pregnancy. Many women have come to me requesting uterine massages during their pregnancies so they will feel connected to their growing babies. But a connection to the baby isn't the only benefit. Awareness of the uterus and all of the physiological changes develops as well. The uterus grows to five times its normal size! It is truly awesome. Gentle uterine massage can help a woman connect not only to her growing baby but also to her growing uterus, and it feels soothing.

Merciér Therapy provides a state of balance during the vital weeks of preconception and throughout pregnancy. In doing so, we are able to make the important mind, heart, and womb connection. Mind—because you are consciously thinking of repair; heart—because you are opening up to love your uterus; and finally you are connecting all three.

Note:

1. Clear Passage Physical Therapy, "Fertility Drugs Increase Thyroid Cancer Risk," www.clearpassage.com/blog/archives/1097.

~5~ *Differences between Holism and Allopathy*

"The greatest mistake in the treatment of diseases is that there are physicians for the body and physicians for the soul, although the two cannot be separated."

—Plato

I have worked for two large and prominent reproductive clinics. In 1993 I was a clinician at a multiple RE clinic in the suburbs of Chicago. I monitored IVF cycles, prepared semen for analysis and IUI, carried out IUI procedures, drew blood, and performed gynecological ultrasounds. I found that work absolutely fascinating. But right off the bat I noticed that many of the doctors would comment on a challenging HSG procedure, embryo transfer, or endometrial biopsy. I started to wonder if each woman had a malpositioned uterus. The only way I could confirm my theory was to chat with one of my favorite doctors. I asked if it were plausible that the reason so many women were not getting pregnant was due to a malposition of the uterus. He looked at me—an undergrad premed student—and said no. I trusted him in the role of teacher, and, knowing that he had a great rapport with his patients, I felt that he answered my question. End of story.

Now that my consciousness had been awakened to the uterus during medical fertility treatment, I was on a mission: to look at each ultrasound and take note while performing an IUI just to see if my thought was guiding me toward something big. My little investigation paid off. I did an off-the-record study and found that many women who came to our clinic had a malposition of the uterus. This means that the uterus was exaggeratedly tilted to the back, front, or one side of the woman's pelvis. Think about the space in the pelvis. There are so many structures that a malposition could negatively affect. Why not work to create the best possible space for conception to occur? As Dr. Jean-Pierre Barral puts it so eloquently, "Lack of proper motion also adversely affects fertility because of failure of the cervix to open and weak vertical movements of the uterus."[1]

I brought my information back to the doctor, and he still did not believe that a malposition would be a contributing factor to a woman's infertility. I continued to place confidence in building a solid, sturdy, strong foundation. What would it hurt? Let's see if it would help women instead of finding my data invalid. That doctor never did look at my thought as valid and still uses medical protocols to help women conceive. His IVF success rate for women ages twenty-five to thirty-eight is 37 percent, according to the SART data submitted for 2005.

I am not happy to report that IVF helps only half of women who seek treatment (about 42 percent across the board). So many factors affect the outcome—age, embryo survival rate, pregnancy transfer rate, number of embryos transferred. In 2000 the *Fertility and Sterility* journal stated this statistic: 600,000 IVF cycles were performed throughout fifty-two countries; 122,000 babies were born. That's a lopsided number. That's 478,000 IVF cycles that resulted in no babies. Why settle for mediocrity?

We are not there yet. With the right preparation, we could most certainly get there. This place that I speak of would shorten the number of cycles, almost without hesitation making that very first cycle a success. It is important to think in this way. Women should not have to endure so many cycles.

Certainly I am not against the medical route for helping couples with their fertility challenges. Some women and men truly need the help of medicine to realize their dream of becoming parents. The problem is that most times allopathic doctors do not want to collaborate with holistic doctors. In fact, the less invasive protocols should be the first route that a couple takes unless a medical risk factor necessitates the help of a medical doctor. My approach is gentle yet effective. There's no need to drive in a thumbtack with a sledgehammer.

Most doctors—who learned in medical school to use drugs, tests, and surgeries to treat people—know standard of care medical protocols, and that is where their knowledge stops. These doctors believe bacteria, viruses, and other foreign microbes are the main causes of disease. Less emphasis is placed on treating parts of the body that are not giving a person trouble, and more is placed on treating the infection, illness, or discomfort. Emphasis on lifestyle change is not very strong.

Fear of the unknown, along with sky-high malpractice, has gotten the best of allopathic doctors, so most are now resistant to change and will not deviate from the medical norm. Here is what I say to that: all women share a common thread—the fact that we are all women; however, we are not all the same. Most IVF and IUI protocols have been written for the use of all women. Being that we all are different, the medical fertility models can be changed ever so slightly to accommodate the needs of women individually. Is the change enough to make the cycle effective in achieving good stimulation, egg retrieval, and embryo transfer? It can be, but this issue goes deeper emotionally than just following a protocol.

Holistic doctors approach your health by looking at you as a whole person—mind, body, and spirit—and prescribing lifestyle, diet, and activity plans that will promote overall health for the long term. They believe that the body contains natural self-healing abilities. Holistic doctors will teach you how to live in such a way that your body heals itself by using natural products and wise lifestyle choices. They consider the main enemies to a healthy life to be toxic chemicals from unnatural products; natural toxins that have built up in the body to an unhealthy proportion; misalignment of skeletal, muscular, or energetic properties in the body; or lifestyle choices that introduce unnatural and unhealthful products and influences into the body. The importance in this model is prevention of illness and proactive living, and most solutions involve using natural products or physical adjustments intended to return the body to its healthy state so the body can heal itself.

Many people choose to use both medical systems in conjunction with one another, seeing a holistic doctor for an overall health plan and turning to an allopathic doctor for assistance with more serious illnesses or diseases when the body seemingly can't fight the problem on its own. Instead of seeing the two medical fields as oppositional, people can take advantage of the benefits of both schools of thought, recognizing that only you know what truly works for your body.

A commitment on your part is most important. To maximize your fertility potential, it is imperative that you work with only one holistic practitioner. I have consulted with couples who were planning to use acupuncture along with my regimen. The combination of more than one holistic practice can be overwhelming and may lead to a conflict of information. Choose one modality and give it all your attention. If you are contemplating IVF, then make sure your physician knows of your intent to use a holistic modality along with the medical IVF protocols. I have to be honest here: many medical doctors will not condone holistic therapy or even know what you are talking about. Their reasons for resistance are many, one being that experience with natural approaches is foreign to them. Medical professionals would rather depend on reading studies. Studies and research are definitely needed when talking about invasive treatments such as drugs and surgery, but research can be skewed and may not show true results.

I choose to use evidence-based references, like testimonials from former clients. It costs several thousands of dollars to conduct a study. As a solo practitioner, I prefer the results that I have observed rather than raise my fees to conduct a study. Sometimes we need to just trust that an alternative or adjunctive modality is valid because we have a comfortable feeling and because other women have found that it worked for them. When women call to tell me they are pregnant or have relief from pain, then that is good enough proof for me.

I have worked with fantastic reproductive endocrinologists. These fertility doctors believe wholeheartedly in the holistic route along with their medical protocols to help create pregnancies. I also have a good rapport with many medical professionals, including nurse practitioners, midwives, physicians, chiropractors, naprapaths, and physical therapists. As I do not practice medicine, I sometimes need to call on these other professionals to make a referral. I would prefer to have good relationships with these folks, because we are all sharing one common goal: helping women. And we all should be playing nice in the sandbox.

Many women come to my practice having already been through the medical route of fertility testing and sometimes treatment. After hysterosalpingograms, endometrial biopsies, blood testing, drug challenges, ultrasounds, artificial ovarian stimulation protocols, oocyte retrieval, embryo transfer . . . failure. All in all, women may feel like the process has been a bit of a circus.

I spent two years working at the fertility clinic, and I learned a lot in that time. We instructed women to call on the first day of their menstrual cycle. Monitoring would start no later than the third cycle day. Appointments were on a first-come, first-served basis, with women needing to arrive at the clinic by 5:30 in the morning. We drew labs and performed ultrasounds. We ordered medications and constructed a schedule in which patients would return for more monitoring. We let women know when to take their HCG injection to trigger ovulation and the time insemination would take place. An IVF cycle process is even more rigorous! Nothing is wrong with these protocols; however, I found myself asking, Why does it have to be so stressful?

Being a patient at a fertility clinic alone is quite different from working with a holistic practitioner alongside a medically oriented protocol.

IVF as a stand-alone regimen

- *○* On the go (rushing to appointments for blood work and ultrasounds)
- *○* Worried about finances (whether insured or uninsured)
- *○* Eating junk food (not instructed otherwise)
- *○* Emotionally out of sorts (lots of drug side effects)
- *○* Hopes much higher than reality (the numbers are there; check for yourself)

IVF and holistic care

- *○* Getting monitored but not rushed (she will learn how to handle and channel stress)
- *○* The financial situation will work itself out (she will learn that it's not about money)
- *○* Eating a clean, nutritious diet (she will be conscious of food choices to ensure and support a healthy first cycle)
- *○* Emotions are in check, she is in check with herself, and she is connected to her heart and womb (excluding drug side effects)
- *○* Hopes are realistic (she has done her homework and is willing to take the chance of the cycle, fully prepared if it does not result in pregnancy)

At the fertility clinic in 1993, the IVF cycle cost somewhere around fourteen thousand dollars. An additional cost to consider was a procedure developed two years earlier called intracytoplasmic sperm injection. During ICSI, an embryologist uses a glass pipette to inject the sperm directly in the oocyte. It is a pretty fascinating procedure but may be linked to the following factors: increased risk of miscarriage, heart problems for affected infants that may require surgery, increased risk of behavioral disorders or learning disabilities, and increased risk of infertility in the woman's children during adulthood. I am not sure if we could really call this a positive medical advancement.

Another procedure is assisted zona hatching, or AZH. The zona is the outer layer of the female oocyte. Sometimes this outer layer is tough for the sperm to penetrate, so an embryologist uses a special solution to rub away that zona. No clinical trial has shown assisted hatching to be beneficial for all patients; in fact, it may be harmful to some patients. However, in certain circumstances it would be beneficial: (1) with frozen embryos (the freeze-thaw process may cause structural changes to the zona); (2) for women older than forty years old; (3) with thickened zona; or (4) after multiple implantation failures.

The costs of ICSI and AZH vary from clinic to clinic. At the clinic that I worked for, couples with no fertility coverage on their insurance plans always looked shell-shocked as new items were added to their ever growing bills. The IVF cycle was no longer an emotional component. The focus shifted quickly to finances, as the clinic wanted its money prior to the egg retrieval. Can you imagine the pressure? I talked with women about how to get creative in paying their bills. Most of them told me they would have done whatever it took to proceed with the cycle. One woman told me that she was in the process of selling her living room and dining room furniture to gather enough money to pay for her fourth round of IVF drugs. She ended up getting pregnant but had no furniture. It is strange that we turn off our normal sense of emotion in order to become pregnant. Making a baby is emotional. Women going through IVF need to be reminded that they are in the process for conception and pregnancy.

It breaks my heart now to take the history of a woman who has undergone one or multiple IVF attempts to no avail. If only she had come to see me prior to her first stimulation cycle. I could have helped her build a solid foundation. A house is built not on a foundation of sand or mud but instead on something much more solid to ensure, from the beginning, the long life of the home.

Let's venture toward some stories from my clinical practice. Enjoy.

Note:

1. Jean-Pierre Barral, Urogenital Manipulation (Vista, CA: Eastland Press, 1993), 143.

Part 2

Case Studies

~6~ *A Malpositioned Uterus*

*"As we struggle to make sense of things,
life looks on in repose."*

—Author unkown

When Kathy and Michael came for a visit, they had already been through a rigorous medical fertility regimen. Nothing medically significant was found to be inhibiting her natural fertility. First was the medical workup and then the suggestion to move toward IVF. Kathy, thirty-two, had a normal FSH and ultrasound, perfectly clear tubes, and no history suggesting risk of disease. Michael had a normal semen analysis and no history of smoking or medical problems.

After discussing possibilities of enduring the IVF cycle, Kathy and Michael agreed that it would be the best way to go. As Kathy says, "I had no idea what we were in for. We just wanted a baby and felt that this would be the quickest route to pregnancy." The schedule read like this: Start birth control pills for one cycle prior to the stimulation process. Start FSH drug to stimulate the ovaries, go in for oocyte or egg retrieval, and finish with the embryo transfer. The first cycle went smoothly with the exception of some general moodiness accompanied by tenderness in the ovaries. Kathy stimulated well and had sixteen follicles retrieved. Eleven embryos resulted, and on the third day, three embryos were transferred. The remaining embryos were frozen and saved for subsequent cycles.

Twelve days after her transfer, Kathy's pregnancy test was negative. Devastated, she and Michael were going to try another cycle. Certainly the next cycle would not be the same, because it would not involve any stimulation or retrieval. With this next cycle the embryologist thawed three more embryos. None of those three survived the process. Three more were then thawed. Two of those were viable and then implanted back into Kathy's uterus. The second cycle resulted in a negative pregnancy test.

Kathy and Michael prepared for the last attempt with her two remaining frozen embryos. Both embryos thawed perfectly—and the third time would be a charm, right? Sadly, the third time resulted in another negative pregnancy test. Kathy was positively beside herself not knowing what to do. Had she done everything she could have done from her perspective? She was certain she had and felt defeated. The couple was encouraged to speak with the reproductive endocrinologist about a new plan. At their appointment, the RE discussed using a different protocol the next time around. Kathy and Michael agreed to take a break from the whole regimen and possibly start all over again a few months later.

So many couples like Kathy and Michael want the quick and easy way to conception and, in the end, find that they are not emotionally prepared. For Kathy and Michael, it took three unsuccessful rounds of IVF to discover that important foundation work needed to be done first.

One of my former clients recommended that Kathy and Michael consult with me. Upon our initial visit we talked thoroughly about her medical and gynecological history. From my standpoint, I was dealing with a woman who had never had any significant medical problems or surgeries. One thing stuck in my mind though—an accident that had occurred while ice-skating as an adult. Kathy had fallen hard on her right hip. I asked her if her embryo transfers had gone smoothly or if there had been a little fidgeting with the catheter upon transfer. She said, "Come to think of it, there was a little trouble getting the catheter into the uterus, and the doctor would get a bit frustrated, telling me that everything was just fine. I never felt any pain or discomfort, but what I did feel was the instrument holding my cervix straight so that the transfer could go smoothly. The doctor used that instrument only for the second and third transfers. I did not notice any problem with the very first transfer. After the procedure was done, I asked why he needed to use that instrument. He told me that my uterus tipped and it was easier to guide the catheter in if he used the tenaculum."

Since Kathy had never experienced any trouble with her menstrual cycles and had no history of infections, I believed Kathy's uterus was malpositioned—and now that idea was confirmed. I also believed she had a progesterone deficiency. Progesterone is an important hormone produced during a woman's cycle. But due to chemical pollutants in our air, water, and soil, our natural hormone production is becoming more and more disrupted. When I have tested women in the luteal phase of their cycle, I have found that progesterone deficiency. This imbalance can be gently corrected using a natural progesterone cream. A small amount of cream is rubbed on the abdomen twice daily after the woman ovulates to help enrich the endometrium and to protect the growing embryo.

I knew exactly what Kathy and I had to do. I tested Kathy's hormone panel and found myriad abnormals that could be fixed using a quality food-based vitamin, thyroid support, and natural progesterone cream in the luteal phase of her cycle. Once she understood her imbalances, we were ready to start pelvic therapy. Pelvic therapy was done three times per week for one month. In one month's time I was able to help her create a connection between her heart and her uterus. She was thinking in a holistic way and even cleaned up her diet to include only organic foods and eliminate soda and caffeine. Within eight weeks after finishing the protocol, Kathy and Michael were expecting their first child. On April 5, 2005, David Michael was born.

The path of holism, education, love, emotional connection, and support was key.

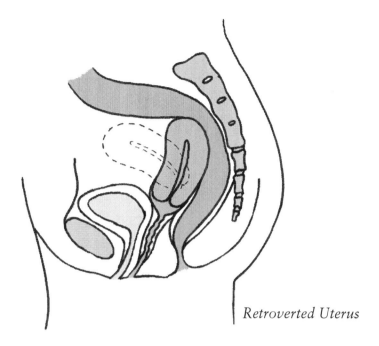

Retroverted Uterus

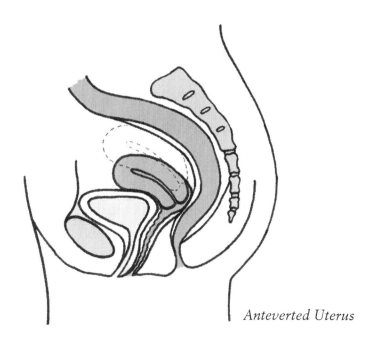

Anteverted Uterus

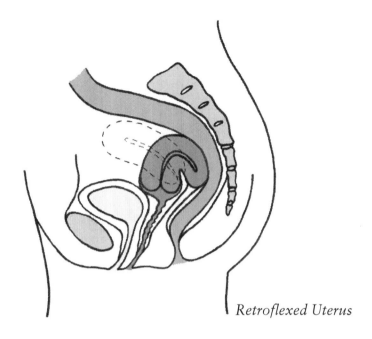

Retroflexed Uterus

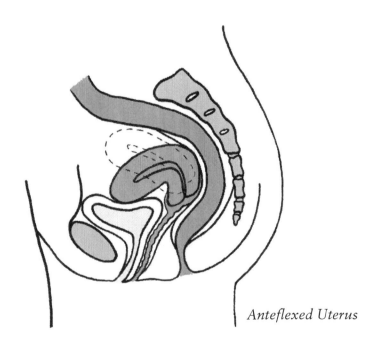

Anteflexed Uterus

~7~ *A Uniquely Shaped Uterus*

"If you can find a path with no obstacles,
it probably doesn't lead anywhere."

—Frank A. Clark

Suzi and Matt came to see me prior to starting their first IVF cycle. Their chiropractor had referred them to me for pelvic therapy and supplement support. Upon our first visit I learned that Suzi had been born with a form of spina bifida that had left her with a misshapen, unicornuate uterus; two noncommunicating fallopian tubes; and two perfectly functioning ovaries.

A unicornuate uterus is a very uncommon condition, affecting only a small percentage of the female population in the U.S. A unicornuate uterus is smaller than a typical uterus and usually has only one functioning fallopian tube. The other side of the uterus may have what is called a rudimentary horn, an underdeveloped "horn" that may or may not be connected to the rest of the uterus and vagina. A fair number of women with a unicornuate uterus have a rudimentary horn.

Suzi and I began with pelvic massage sessions three times per week for four weeks. Within that time Suzi was beginning to connect with her uterus.

With each session I could feel the uterus becoming more mobile. Anything that is living has to be able to move freely. No organism should be stuck in one place, otherwise it is losing its life.

As our work progressed, blood flow increased to the uterus and ovaries, therefore increasing the chances of a productive stimulation cycle. Suzi's stimulation cycle started once we completed her pelvic therapy regimen. But her RE overstimulated her, resulting in a trip to the emergency room, no egg retrieval, and no pregnancy. Suzi and Matt decided they were not getting the care they needed, so I supported them in choosing to switch to another care provider.

The process to change REs involved Suzi picking up her frozen embryos and moving them to her new doctor's embryology facility. Matt and Suzi were feeling confident with their choice to change providers. Under the care of her new physician and starting her second IVF cycle, she finally felt at ease yet still a bit nervous.

In preparation for her embryo transfer, Suzi and I worked together to ensure a favorable environment within her pelvis. Her transfer was scheduled, and together we prepared her uterus for a flawless transfer. Ten days after her transfer, Suzi and Matt found out that she was pregnant.

We continued working together to help Suzi prepare for a healthy pregnancy and birth. I saw her once a month to check the ligaments and muscles in the pelvis and lower back. I believe her pregnancy went so beautifully due to many factors, including being conscious of her diet, receiving regular bodywork, and focusing on a healthy state of mind.

At thirty-seven weeks Suzi had a lovely vaginal birth. Their baby boy was born of more than adequate size and in excellent health. This was a case that truly needed a medically assisted reproductive intervention. Happily, Suzi and Matt have decided to endure the rigors of another IVF cycle. This is the only way for them to conceive, and they wish for at least one more biological child.

Suzi and Matt are now pursuing their second IVF attempt. In preparation for this new cycle, we did some follow-up pelvic massages to ensure a positive stimulation cycle. Sure enough, her first cycle produced twenty-six eggs at retrieval.

~8~ *Postsurgical Scar Tissue*

"Healing is a matter of time, but it is sometimes also a matter of opportunity."

—Hippocrates

Tracey had been seeing a reproductive endocrinologist for one year. Throughout that year each medically assisted attempt failed. At first this thirty-seven-year old was told that she needed to undergo the typical battery of tests to determine the source of her fertility challenges.

Test after subsequent test revealed nothing of significance. Her husband's semen analysis was normal. Due to Tracey's age, the physician strongly suggested going directly to IVF. Uncomfortable with IVF, they decided to try gonadotropin stimulating drugs along with IUI. The doctor advised that this would be the less invasive path but may improve Tracey and her husband's chances to conceive by only 15 percent. After six unsuccessful IUI cycles, they decided to move to IVF.

Tracey was not settled with the decision to move forward with IVF but knew that she wanted a baby. All she thought about was getting pregnant and taking the prescribed regimen of suppression and stimulation drugs to prepare for her egg retrieval. Paying careful attention to her calendar, she moved her way through the first stimulation cycle. At times Tracey felt depressed and angry that she and her husband had resorted to that route of assistance.

By the time her ovaries were ready for retrieval, she had ten follicles that measured 20–24 mm. Intracytoplasmic sperm injection was performed on all ten ovum, and seven of the embryos became viable. On the third day three embryos were transferred. The uterine lining was optimal and Tracey was started on progesterone injections. Twelve days after her transfer, she went in for her first pregnancy test, and it was negative. Tracey was crushed, as she had gone into the cycle feeling ready to endure the protocol of drugs, ultrasounds, and blood tests.

No one had worked with Tracey to prepare her for the emotional roller coaster that typically comes with an IVF cycle. She trusted her doctor to inform her about every aspect of the cycle, and with that thinking she believed she needed to do something different with her next cycle. As the next cycle started, she promised herself to attend yoga classes and make minor dietary changes. Mind you, her diet was not good to begin with. Tracey picked up a book about what to eat while trying to improve fertility. Tracey's intentions were good, but she made it to only one yoga class and did not change anything about her diet. After her second and third IVF attempts failed, she decided not to go through another cycle.

One month after finishing her third cycle, Tracey called me for a consult. I started by obtaining Tracey's complete history. I appreciated her candidness when talking with me. We spoke about her feelings regarding the IVF cycles. She told me that those cycles were some of the most physically difficult and emotionally trying times because she had not felt well prepared. I asked her what she thought she needed to be better prepared for IVF. She said she felt rushed and like just another number while going through the process. For instance, Tracey had called to ask questions and sometimes never got a return call. She was disappointed.

At that point in our visit I had Tracey empty her bladder. Once she had done so, I asked her to lie on my table so I could assess the position of her uterus and condition of the surrounding musculature. I was just floored by what I saw! This poor woman had told me about her previous history of a routine appendectomy (the only thing that arose with her medical and surgical history), but I never expected such a large incision. What had started out as routine surgery had turned into a nightmare. Once the surgeon had removed her appendix, twenty-four hours later Tracey experienced severe abdominal pain. The surgeon had to reopen Tracey's abdomen and discovered that a massive blood clot had formed after the original surgery. The incision for the second surgery was a long, vertical line that started just below the xiphoid process and ended just above the pubic bone. Tracey's belly looked like it had been cinched together from side to side. That was by far the largest abdominal incision I had ever seen.

I started to palpate around on her abdomen and pelvis, finding that nearly all of the structures below the skin's surface were completely stuck together. It's no wonder Tracey's bowel movements were few and far between and that she had not conceived. The restrictions were advanced, and there was little if any movement within the organ structures. Try to do a push-up with your arms stuck at your sides. That is how all of her abdominal organs had been functioning since her surgery.

We worked and worked on the adhesions, trying to free up the muscles, ligaments, and organs. It took many sessions to be able to palpate results but only a few sessions for Tracey to feel a sense of freeness. It's not surprising that her numerous IVF cycles failed. If her reproductive doctor had known anything about the damage that scar tissue can cause within the pelvis, then maybe she would have used caution when approaching IVF. And if her doctor had known of the soft tissue release work that could have prepared Tracey, then she could have referred her patient to the most appropriate care provider and seen a successful response to the IVF cycles. Perhaps with the proper restriction release of all the scar tissue, a patient would not need assistance from a medical provider and instead would become pregnant on her own.

Tracey finished my Shared Journey protocol in March 2010. She is still patiently waiting, taking all of the prescribed herbs and progesterone cream and learning about the new connection with herself that she has discovered with Merciér Therapy. I wish her all the best and hope she will continue to be patient during her journey.

~9~ Anxiety While Trying to Conceive

"Fear is the lengthened shadow of ignorance."

—Arnold Glasow

Recently a thirty-two-year-old woman came to see me for help with a fertility challenge. From our initial visit I could tell that Lisa was anxious. Her anxiety felt contagious, as I started to wonder if I could work with her. Lisa's ob-gyn had told her to wait until she missed a period and then to call her office. When Lisa never missed her period and never got any solid answers on why she was not getting pregnant, she came to see me.

I started by obtaining Lisa's medical history. Nothing raised any red flags. She had a history of one natural pregnancy that ended in a miscarriage at ten weeks. We talked for two hours as I recorded each and every detail of her cycles since her menarche. Sounded to me like Lisa had symptoms of anxiety, luteal phase progesterone insufficiency, and a malpositioned uterus.

I suggested a protocol of herbs, vitamins, natural progesterone, and pelvic massage therapy. Lisa was a compliant client. Diligently she returned three times per week for one month. And knowing Lisa's history, I knew she was eating a healthful diet, not smoking or drinking alcohol, exercising regularly, and taking her supportive supplements.

But Lisa, I gathered, was angry with herself for her miscarriage. We talked about why miscarriage happens and that she was not the responsible cause. I started to believe that her anxiety was causing her inability to become pregnant. There was only so much I could help her with, so we worked on relaxing during each pelvic therapy session. In our work together Lisa learned that she was disconnected from her womb. So I asked her to lie in bed each night, prior to sleeping, with her hands on her lower abdomen to be able to hear what her body was telling her. Once she was comfortable with that type of listening, it became apparent to her that her womb was asking for forgiveness.

Forgiving her uterus was the start of something new for her. Lisa had never been asked to think in such a different way as that. The groundwork had been initiated and an empowering energy surrounded her each time we talked. She had taken a less controlling approach to her fertility and was allowing herself time for mindful thoughts.

I really believed that together Lisa and I had made some headway with her thinking about fertility. After completing our work, I learned that Lisa had decided to consult with an RE. She had not given herself enough time to process what she had just learned. Only two weeks after she left me, she had an appointment with her RE. Lisa underwent a battery of tests including lab work, ultrasound, HSG, and endometrial biopsy. All of her tests came back as nonconclusive of having any medical pathologies or problems. I do know her RE, and he told me that her uterus was very mobile.

Experts estimate that upwards of 80 percent of fertility issues are stress related. Perhaps nothing ages us faster, internally and externally, than high stress. While eliminating anxiety and pressure altogether in this fast-paced world may be idealistic, massage can, without a doubt, help manage stress. This translates into decreased anxiety, enhanced sleep quality, greater energy, improved concentration, increased circulation, and reduced fatigue. Clients often report a sense of perspective and clarity after receiving a massage. The emotional balance that bodywork provides can often be just as vital and valuable as the more tangible physical benefits.

Research continues to show the enormous benefits of touch—ranging from treating chronic diseases, neurological disorders, and injuries to alleviating the tensions of modern lifestyles. Consequently, the medical community is actively embracing bodywork, and massage is becoming an integral part of fertility care.

Many women deny themselves the opportunity to take a less aggressive approach to their fertility. When I say less aggressive, I mean more time for reflection and less time for worry. Relaxation needs to be added to this critical time of creation.

In the end, Lisa never did become pregnant. Hers was a case of not being awake to her own intuition and ability to learn about herself. She had a tremendous disconnect with her body. Creation of life may be imminent but cannot easily happen if you cannot meet yourself in the middle.

~10~ A Lovely Surprise

"Don't tell people how to do things. Tell them what to do and let them surprise you with their results."

—George S. Patton

Carrie and her husband, Kris, came to see me for a fertility consult after reading my practice information on my Web site. While gathering information, I noticed that they lived in Wisconsin. My practice is in South Elgin, Illinois. Determined to start care with me, Carrie made the commitment to drive from Wisconsin to Illinois for the Shared Journey Fertility Program.

I listened to Carrie's history during her first visit, and her menstrual cycles seemed normal—bleeding every twenty-eight to thirty days with no significant clotting or cramping. The only unusual thing I noticed was that Carrie sometimes bled for six days then started up again on day seven. She had never had surgery; therefore, minimal if any scar tissue presented in the pelvis and abdominal viscera. Her medical history was negative of any autoimmune diseases or abnormal pathologies. Carrie was not a smoker nor was she on any pharmaceuticals. Kris underwent a semen analysis, and no abnormalities were found. Why would it be difficult for a woman so healthy to become pregnant?

Continuing to assemble information, I found that four years prior she had tried using the drug Clomid for five nonconsecutive cycles to no avail. Carrie's doctor did no monitoring during the use of the drug, so I could not determine how she stimulated with Clomid.

When using a drug such as Clomid, the patient needs to be monitored by ultrasound and blood levels to be sure she is responding favorably and not under- or overstimulating. Also, it is helpful to know when ovulation is occurring or going to occur by good measurement of the follicles. Ultrasound can be a helpful tool in discerning ovulatory timing, as Clomid will change the sticky ovulatory mucus and may cloud the woman's own self-monitoring.

In general, Clomid dries out the vagina and endometrium, leaving the vagina even more acidic than usual. Keep in mind that the normal, healthy vaginal ecosystem is acidic, but the acidity kills sperm. That is why the semen that accompanies the sperm is alkaline. The semen transiently protects the sperm in the vagina until they can move safely past the cervical mucus into the uterus and tubes. Sperm left behind (usually because of poor motility) are pretty much destroyed by the vaginal acidity in five minutes, so they have to be quick. In fact, the quickest sperm can be found in the tube within ninety seconds of being deposited in the vagina.

It is helpful to couple intrauterine insemination with Clomid to ensure the best outcome for each cycle. By inseminating the sperm directly into the uterus, they are given the best chance of survival right out of the gate. Insemination injects the washed sperm directly into the uterus and completely bypasses the hostility of the vaginal environment altogether, therefore increasing the chances of pregnancy with each cycle.

One week after her first appointment, Carrie arrived at my office to start pelvic therapy. We agreed to see each other for four condensed sessions once a week lasting ninety minutes each. (A therapy session is usually thirty to forty minutes in length.) Upon my initial palpation of her uterus, I noticed that the pelvic ligaments on the right side were tightened, pulling the uterus into the right ilium (hip bone) and making the entire left side of the pelvis very lengthened—meaning there was a lot of room in one side and practically none in the opposite side. Carrie tolerated the therapy well, and as we finished our session I appreciated that the midline position of the uterus was much more flexible and moving more fluid. The tightness was still noted but much better.

When our second session started, I noticed that Carrie's uterus had stayed in the same position from our first session. She felt a sense of freeness and increased movement within her pelvis. That session was uneventful and produced the same great results as the last. The uterine ligaments were now like rubber bands instead of tightly pulled rope.

The third session was cycle day one of her menstrual cycle. I worked as intensely as I had with the prior sessions due to her negative history of endometriosis. Women with endometriosis should not have intense pelvic work done during menses because the endometrial implants bleed as well during the menses and could spread the cellular components of endometriosis around the peritoneum. This can lead to increased and intense pain.

Carrie had noticed that day one of this period was different. She was experiencing pain and had to take ibuprofen. I encouraged her to do so to help decrease the inflammatory response. As we continued our work, I used a slightly lighter touch to begin our session. Once the ibuprofen took effect, I started to work deeper. Carrie was able to tolerate the session just fine.

Our last treatment was uneventful and produced no pain. I told Carrie to continue her herbal regimen and to periodically let me know how she was doing. Once the six-month period post-therapy was completed and if no pregnancy occurred, then we were to regroup and discuss additional sessions.

I am happy to say that Carrie and Kris conceived at nearly the six-month post-therapy mark. I commend Carrie for following her heart and staying true to the therapy and herbal regimen. It is a conscious choice to be patient with oneself while trying to conceive. Carrie is now ten weeks pregnant and has chosen to birth their baby at home with the skilled wisdom of a midwife.

~11~ *Pelvic Organ Mobility*

"'Uncertainty will always be part of the taking charge process' [Harold Geneen]. Most times it is worthwhile to do nothing."

—Jennifer Merciér

My friend is a smart internal medicine physician who is able to appreciate the integrative holistic approach. He encouraged his friend who is also in the profession of allopathic medicine to come see me for help with a fertility challenge.

During her first visit, Manisha, a twenty-nine-year-old physical therapist in a hospital system, told me about her medical and gynecological history. As we talked, the only significance with her past was chronic anemia and varicose veins in her legs.

Manisha and her husband, Agit, had been trying to conceive for well over a year and had chosen to see a reproductive endocrinologist prior to seeing me. Her menstrual cycles were every twenty-six to twenty-eight days with no pain and no gynecological pathologies. Her cycle day three follicular-stimulating hormone was 9.8, and she complained of no pain during her menses. Her RE, finding nothing wrong with Manisha, suggested a diagnostic laparoscopy to see if they were indeed missing something. In the end, the RE told the couple that structurally the uterus and ovaries looked normal and that nothing abnormal was seen. However, Manisha's pelvic ligaments were tightened while the surgery was taking place. Why? No reason was given. One predominant reason to tighten pelvic ligaments is in the case of pelvic organ prolapse. She had not experienced organ prolapse.

My work was clear-cut. I knew that we had to enable pelvic organ mobility. This made plenty of sense to Manisha, who herself works with patients to restore function in certain areas of the body. However, she had never heard of the type of therapy I was performing.

Moving forward, we condensed the therapy into six one-hour sessions. During the first session, Manisha's uterus was pulled so taught that I noted hardly any movement at all. The uterus was in a slightly anteflexed position (exaggerated position to the front of the pelvis). Our first session released many trigger points within the surrounding musculature and ligamentous structures. I started her on the herbal fertility protocol and supported her thyroid and sent her on her way.

The next session was cycle day two for Manisha. She was not complaining of any residual pain from our last treatment, and her period came early on cycle day twenty-four. This was unusual for her but not unusual for a woman undergoing such intense pelvic manipulation therapy. Suspecting a luteal phase deficiency, I added a natural progesterone cream to her regimen. She was to use the progesterone cream topically on cycle days fourteen through twenty-eight. Progesterone must be used once ovulation is suspected, or it can actually impede natural ovulation.

By her third treatment, Manisha noticed discomfort on her left ovary. That was cycle day twelve. A follicle was probably growing on the ovary, causing a full feeling. We continued our session without a problem.

In our fourth treatment, cycle day sixteen, Manisha noticed an increase in fertile cervical mucus. Sure enough, an LH surge was present, and I instructed the couple to have intercourse that evening and the following day.

The fifth treatment was the fourth day of a new cycle. It was okay that Manisha had not conceived with the last cycle; the couple understood that the process of conception requires patience. We continued our work, and I could feel mobility within the pelvic organs. It was an amazing shift from our first session.

Our last and final session was her cycle day ten. Manisha was quite aware of the signs of ovulation by then and went on her way with the prescribed supplements and progesterone. She was feeling great and, I think, a little skeptical. One month after finishing our sessions, Manisha called to let me know that her period was a few days late and that she had taken a pregnancy test. The test was positive. According to Manisha's last menstrual period, she was five weeks pregnant.

Manisha had an uneventful pregnancy and went on to deliver a healthy baby girl.

"As a physical therapist, my daily practice involves creating an individualized treatment plan for each patient by choosing the right techniques for treatment and correct assessment of impairments. So my husband and I were understandably frustrated when after consulting with various doctors and undergoing numerous medical tests (which were all basically normal), we were told that we basically had two options—that we could keep trying for an indefinite time or pursue IUI/IVF. We had already been trying for a while and were not comfortable with the second option, since our medical testing had not shown any problems to warrant that treatment. Our answer came when a mutual doctor friend brought Jennifer into our lives, who looked at the holistic picture. We realized that I was literally in the right hands! As a physical therapist, I know how musculoskeletal imbalances can lead to pain and dysfunction, but didn't realize the tightness and imbalances I had until Jennifer performed her pelvic massage techniques and felt immediate relief physically and mentally! We became pregnant right after the completion of our treatment with

Jennifer, and ever since, I have been free of severely painful menstrual cycles. Jennifer helped give my husband and me our greatest joy of being parents to our beautiful child!"

—Manisha Patel, physical therapist

~12~ Endometriosis

"Attitude is a little thing that makes a big difference."

—Winston Churchill

An all too often diagnosis of endometriosis has surfaced in the last several years. While the cause of the disease is not certain, many speculations exist. One belief is that a retrograde of endometrial cells may be present. These cells, normally inside the uterus, start to flow backward out of the fallopian tubes and into the abdominal cavity. These cells grow and flourish due to the presence of hormones and the menstrual cycle. Once the cells inhabit the space, they bleed and form adhesive tissue on the uterus, ovaries, bladder, bowel, rectum, and other tissues. These endometrial implants can become very aggressive, causing pain and abnormalities of the pelvic tissues.

Endometriosis can cause infertility due to scar tissue impeding ovulation and can create tubal problems. Hormones and menstrual irregularities due to this disease can also play a role. Endometriosis is not a surgical disease; surgery will not cure it. However, surgical laparoscopy is the only way endometriosis can be diagnosed. Once the diagnosis is confirmed, a regimen of drugs may be prescribed to keep the symptoms at rest. Future surgeries may become necessary to improve fertility, manage pain, remove endometriomas, and ablate adhesions.

Endometriosis affects over one million women yearly in the U.S. While most cases are diagnosed in women twenty-five to thirty-five years old, endometriosis has been reported in girls as young as eleven. The disease is rare in postmenopausal women and is more commonly found in white women than African-American and Asian women. Delaying pregnancy until an older age is also believed to increase the risk of developing endometriosis.

Many of my fertility clients either have symptoms of endometriosis or a confirmed diagnosis of the disease. I suggest an aggressive herbal tincture along with luteal phase natural progesterone cream to help combat the painful symptoms. The herbal formula helps eliminate the endometrial cells naturally, and during this process I would not use any pelvic therapy in order to not stir up any of those shedding cells. I think of this time as a preparation for the physical work.

The next phase, consisting of the pelvic massage sessions, can bring extreme relaxation and healing. The therapy helps create the important connection that only a woman can make with herself. By the fourth session she is feeling great relief and many times will start to feel taller too. I know, it sounds a little crazy, but releasing that tight scar tissue creates a lengthening of musculature. A sense of freeness and well-being occurs. Women are not free of the disease but have made a good decision to take a gentle route to helping themselves.

I met Kelly, age thirty-six, when she was suffering from pelvic pain due to stage four endometriosis. Her history included six laparoscopies and various drug treatments to keep her symptoms at bay. Due to severe adhesions, scar tissue, and a nonfunctioning right ovary, Kelly's gynecologist told her to never expect to become pregnant. That information was not relevant though, being that she was coming to see me for help with control of pain and discomfort. Kelly, who had never been pregnant, had no urgency to conceive.

Upon our first visit, I noted a good bit of restriction within her abdomen and pelvis. Kelly's gait was suggesting a tilt on her pelvis and a torsion within her ribcage, all caused by her numerous surgical procedures. From there I formulated a nice protocol for her. We started our work together, and it produced a small bit of discomfort. Keep in mind that if an organ, muscle, ligament, fascia, or other tissue holds a pattern long enough, that position becomes normal. It could be the wrong position, but ultimately the body compensates and starts to function abnormally. Keeping aware of your posture and movement patterns will give your body the best chance to set into a normal functioning place.

Kelly canceled her second visit due to pelvic discomfort. I encouraged her to use a moist heating pad to help with the relief of inflammation. Ultimately I suggested that she come back in to continue the regimen. She agreed that after her pain had dissipated she did feel a certain level of freeness. During our second visit I noticed more mobility within the pelvis. It was slight, but nonetheless it was something. The day after our session, Kelly called and told me that no other modality of therapeutic work had been so tangible.

By her third visit we were well on our way to bringing about some real relief to her endometriosis pain. In the past it had been recommended that she use prescription pain medicine. The pain medicine made her feel tired and caused many unwanted side effects that made her job as a teacher difficult. So we worked diligently to cause a change within her pelvic tilt and rib cage torsion. By just following a pelvic massage regimen, we were able to free up fascial restrictions and create balance within the space. I felt confident in the progress of our work.

Fast-forward to session twelve. Kelly was feeling so good that she was ready to enlist in yoga classes, continue to take the supportive herbs, and use progesterone cream. I saw so many wonderful changes within this woman and knew I had helped her positively impact her view of her journey to wellness.

Twelve weeks later I received a call from Kelly. It was a Sunday morning and she called from a drugstore where she had just purchased a pregnancy test. Not waiting until she got home, she took the test in the store. It was positive. That result was a true defiance of what her doctor had suggested. She was in shock. I advised her to go home, relax, and think about how she felt. According to her last period, she was already six weeks along.

Kelly called her doctor. He was in complete disbelief and asked her to come in for a blood level to confirm. Sure enough, it was positive. An ultrasound was then ordered to see if her pregnancy was growing in her uterus. Sometimes when so much scar tissue is present, a tubal malfunction can displace the embryo from implanting within the uterus, making it ectopic. Kelly's pregnancy was in her uterus.

Women with this aggressive disease have many options with a combination of holistic therapies and conventional medicine. Correction is possible with proper balances of nutrition, herbs, site specific pelvic therapy, and a sound emotional state.

"Endometriosis is a difficult condition which is often poorly diagnosed, poorly understood and poorly treated. As Western doctors we have to admit our shortcomings and trust qualified and experienced complementary practitioners."

—Dr. Michael Dooley, gynecologist

Dorset County Hospital, London

~13~ Secondary Infertility After a C-Section

*"A bend in the road is not the end of the road...
unless you fail to make the turn."*

—Author Unkown

Cesarean sections can cause countless troubles for the future health of women. If a C-section is warranted for medical reasons, then by all means it needs to be done. It can be a lifesaving procedure for both mother and baby. All too often, though, C-sections are performed for convenience. Whether emergent or elective, a C-section brings common psychological outcomes of negative feelings, fear, guilt, anger, and postpartum depression. Question any reason a doctor gives you for a C-section.

According to the International Cesarean Awareness Network, a C-section should be necessary only in the following situations:

- Complete placenta previa at term
- Transverse lie at complete dilation
- Prolapsed cord
- Abrupted placenta
- Eclampsia or HELLP syndrome with failed induction of labor

- Large uterine tumor that blocks the cervix at complete dilation (Most fibroids will move upward as the cervix opens, moving it out of baby's path.)
- True fetal distress confirmed with a fetal scalp sampling or biophysical profile
- True absolute cephalopelvic disproportion
- Initial outbreak of active herpes at the onset of labor
- Uterine rupture[1]

Half of all women who undergo C-sections suffer complications, including infection, blood loss and hemorrhage, hysterectomy, transfusions, bladder and bowel injury, incisional endometriosis, heart and lung complications, blood clots in the legs, anesthesia complications, and rehospitalization due to surgical complications. That's not to mention the mother's possible psychological and emotional trauma. Scar tissue adhesions pose the potential for chronic complications of pelvic pain, bowel problems, and pain during sexual intercourse. Scar tissue also makes subsequent C-sections more difficult to perform, increasing a woman's risk of injury to her organs. Approximately 180 women in the U.S. die annually from elective repeat cesareans, and the mortality rate for women who undergo just one C-section is two to four times that of women who give birth vaginally.[2]

On more than a dozen occasions I have worked with women who suffer from secondary infertility due to prior C-section scar tissue. Although millions of women are affected by the painful experience of secondary infertility (the inability to become pregnant or to carry a pregnancy to term following the birth of one or more children), it generally remains unacknowledged and is an invisible condition.

During the initial session of pelvic massage with a woman who has endured a C-section, I typically feel a tight band of scar tissue in the lower abdomen. This scar tissue is fibrous and tough on the superficial layer but also is the same underneath the skin. Most times the scar tissue acts like glue under the surface of the abdomen's muscle layer. It can affect all of the structures surrounding the healing uterus.

I encourage women to move forward with twelve pelvic massage therapy sessions to help break down those fibrous adhesions of scar tissue. I have never seen anything but healthy repair of the lower pelvic area.

Case in point: A woman named Cindy visited me. She had a two-year-old son born by a necessary cesarean. She had been trying with her husband for almost a year to conceive a second time.

Cindy's son sees a pediatrician in my office building. After hearing of Cindy's disappointment month after month, the pediatrician told her to see me for help. I remember our first visit; Cindy was skeptical of the therapy. Upon palpation of her scar, I noticed an immovability within her superficial skin. While working through the layers of tissue, I could feel the fixation within her pelvic organs and surrounding structures. Layer by layer I was able to implement much needed movement back into the musculature and ligaments. Soon thereafter, the uterus followed suit.

I asked Cindy to see me twice a week. She complied. After just eight weeks Cindy was pregnant. She carried her baby to thirty-eight weeks and at her doctor's urging had a repeat cesarean. Cindy and her husband plan on not having more children.

Each time a woman endures subsequent C-sections, the risks become much higher. My intention is to ensure that women are well informed to make a good decision prior to electing for a surgical birth. If it is medically necessary, there really are no other options. Once the C-section surgery is done, realize that your pelvis needs to have soft tissue therapy to properly rehabilitate.

By just addressing the uterus itself, the result is always positive.

Notes:

1. International Cesarean Awareness Network, www.ican-online.org/pregnancy/cesarean-fact-sheet.

2. Ibid.

~14~ Uterine Prolapse

"Healing takes courage, and we all have courage, even if we have to dig a little to find it."

—Tori Amos

In our first meeting, Wendy told me she had experienced seven home births and was currently twelve weeks pregnant with baby number eight. Wendy's midwife for baby number seven had pulled on her umbilical cord and caused a prolapse of her uterus. Prior to her seventh birth, Wendy had no troubles at all. I asked how she knew there was a problem. Wendy told me she could feel her cervix coming out of her vagina and that intercourse felt different. She was not feeling pain; just the fact that the uterus was hanging so low troubled her.

I started doing manual soft tissue therapeutic work on her round ligaments, uterus, and sacrum. We saw each other once a week for the entire pregnancy. Wendy was committed to regaining strength in her womb and surrounding structures to help ensure the safe delivery of baby number eight. Along with the manual work, I suggested that she buy a Belly Bandit for support. The Belly Bandit company will tell you not to wear its product during pregnancy. I am sure this is a disclaimer on the company's part. Make sure you buy the correct size and wear it only for support. The Belly Bandit should provide gentle support for your growing uterus and lower back.

At forty weeks into her pregnancy, Wendy started labor. Her midwife told her that the only way she could deliver at home was in a birthing tub. The water pressure in the birthing tub would keep her internal organs high in her pelvis and provide positive gravity for her heavy uterus. The birth of the baby would be gentle and gradual, with no pulling or tugging on her baby's umbilical cord. After only three hours of labor, Wendy gave birth to a healthy six pound nine ounce baby girl. The placenta delivered on its own into the birthing tub twenty minutes after the birth. Once Wendy got out of the tub and showered, she was examined and learned that the cervix was no longer protruding into the vagina. She was instructed to continue wearing her Belly Bandit for support.

Wendy came in at six weeks postpartum to continue receiving pelvic massage therapy. It has been four years since the birth, and all is still going well with no signs of prolapse. I fully believe that women need to take charge of their care to bring about the best outcome. Wendy was committed to following a regimen to ensure a healthy pregnancy and birth. I have a great deal of respect for that kind of commitment.

~15~ *Uterine Fibroids*

"Change always comes bearing gifts."

—Price Pritchett

I first saw Kara for a consult when she was twelve weeks and six days pregnant with her first baby. Kara's chiropractic physician referred her to me to check the mobility of the uterus and the ligaments in relationship to the fibroids. Upon my gathering information of current happenings, she mentioned some episodes of moderate to heavy bleeding during the pregnancy. To be precise, she complained of six different episodes with no blood clots noted.

Kara brought in an ultrasound photo that had been taken just a few days earlier. The bleed around the pregnancy could be seen predominantly, yet the baby looked well and was of adequate growth.

I proceeded to get the rest of Kara's medical and gynecological history. She had a low hemoglobin level of nine, probably due to her recent occurrence of uterine bleeding. Her medical history was clear of any abnormal pathologies. Her recent gynecological history included a few uterine fibroids and regular menstrual cycles.

Uterine fibroids are noncancerous tumors consisting of fibers or fibrous tissue that arise in the uterus. They are the most common growth of the female genital tract. These tumors are highly sensitive to estrogen. They develop following the onset of menstruation, enlarge during pregnancy, decrease, and often disappear after menopause, when estrogen levels decrease by half. They can be as small as a hen's egg or, commonly, grow to the size of an orange or grapefruit. The largest fibroid on record weighed over one hundred pounds. Uterine fibroids afflict many women, especially from age thirty-five to fifty. One in five women in the U.S. has at least some evidence of fibroids. Discovery is usually accidental and is coincidental with heavier periods, irregular bleeding, or painful periods. Fibroids will not disappear once discovered, but they can shrink based on diet and use of the correct dose of natural progesterone.

As I started to palpate and navigate my way around Kara's pelvis, I noticed that her uterus measured much larger than a twelve-week pregnancy. I am a midwife and have measured hundreds of pregnant bellies at various times throughout pregnancy. Kara's uterus had surpassed any other palpation I had ever felt. The measurement was that of a sixteen-week-size uterus.

The work I did was very gentle not to disturb the delicate situation, and I felt it unnecessary to work on the uterus itself. I found that her uterus was tilted exaggeratedly to the left, while the fibroid was felt at the height of the fundus (top of the uterus). I worked only on Kara's ligaments, surrounding pelvic musculature, and into her hip joints. She said that the therapy felt pleasant and did not create any pain.

In conclusion to our first visit I suggested that Kara start topical progesterone cream each day along with Floradix to help replace the iron she had lost due to the recent bleeding episodes. We agreed to see each other for a follow-up in two weeks and to continue with pelvic therapy two times per month until she delivered.

Kara called me two weeks later to say she had miscarried the pregnancy at fifteen weeks.

We followed up at eight weeks postmiscarriage. Kara was feeling pretty good and ready to start a twelve-session regimen of Merciér Therapy. Prior to the start of therapy, she had an ultrasound to measure her fibroids.

Her fibroids were palpable immediately. Shrinking and softening those areas in the uterus is what we had to work toward. Kara wanted to get pregnant again, but this next time she wanted to ensure that she would not miscarry. Progesterone was started in the luteal phase of her cycle, but only after ovulation. Remember, if used incorrectly, progesterone can actually inhibit ovulation. On the sixth treatment she came in with an ultrasound report. One of the larger fibroids measured 5 cm. Diligently Kara came in three times per week for one month for some intense work.

No pain or abnormal bleeding was noted during treatment. Another ultrasound checked the size of that larger 5 cm fibroid, finding that it had shrunk to 2 cm.

Menses commenced as usual, uneventfully. Kara finished her sessions at the end of July and conceived again in August. Her daughter was born in May at forty-plus weeks. The vaginal delivery was lovely and uneventful.

~16~ Sexual Abuse Trauma

"Forgiving does not erase the bitter past. A healed memory is not a deleted memory. Instead, forgiving what we cannot forget creates a new way to remember. We change the memory of our past into a hope for our future."

—Lewis B. Smedes

Medicine has been on a downhill slope in taking care of us for some time now. Again, let me be clear that not all medical professionals are ill-intended, and we do need them in medical crises. However, medical treatments such as testing, pharmaceuticals, and surgery are widely overused. Patients are becoming medically mismanaged and lost in our politically and financially driven medical system.

Case in point: A forty-year-old woman visited me to talk about how Merciér Therapy may be therapeutic given her problem. In my gathering her history, she mentioned many names of physicians, therapists, and counselors who had all seen her for her history of sexual abuse and pelvic pain. She had tried numerous medications, including injections into trigger points in her vaginal walls. One physician even suggested a vaginoplasty. A vaginoplasty is a reconstructive surgery used to construct or reconstruct a vaginal canal and mucous membrane. Why would that have been a viable suggestion? The surgery would probably have caused more trouble and created scar tissue that would have further displaced the tissue of her introitus.

Not one of those medical professionals suggested any type of holistic modality. Indeed, that was just what she needed. A change in course is necessary when medicine fails so miserably and brings no relief to the suffering patient.

Upon our first visit I learned of a tragic event that occurred when Linda was a young nine years old and continued well into her teenage years. A male in this woman's family had penetrated her vagina with an object time and time again. As an adult, she suffered from great emotional pain, as well as physical pain within her pelvis. She fully understood that a pill was not going to fulfill her need for healing. In essence, her healing never began because she had been passed from one medical doctor and therapist to another. Linda told me she had wasted so much time trying to find her healing path and did not know the resources with which to find a helpful and well-trained holistic professional. She had tried massage therapy, acupuncture, hypnotherapy, exercise, a nutritionist, and yoga—all which provided temporary relief but did not entirely address her pain.

I suggested that we start with a series of Merciér soft tissue therapeutic pelvic sessions. At first Linda was skeptical because she had never heard of any therapy like that, and it meant she would have to let me address her abdomen and pelvis. Typically we women guard our abdomens as places of safeness. When a woman has a massage treatment, the therapist rarely, if ever, does any abdominal work. I have had over one hundred professional and student massages, and none of them have ever addressed my abdomen. When I asked my most recent massage therapist if she would do some abdominal work, she was shocked that I had even asked. She told me that she does not work in that region and that most women she has worked with have been adamant about not touching their abdomens. This makes me wonder if perhaps many women have been inappropriately touched or abused in their lifetimes.

Linda and I completed her first session at her first visit. She was nervous. I told her that she was the boss. If she wanted me to stop our session, then she needed to let me know. We did end up stopping the therapy a few times. Our first session took ninety minutes—sixty minutes longer than a usual session. I did not mind at all. I knew I could help her and would give of my time as she needed. As we worked, she was feeling pain in her vagina. I asked if it was okay to continue, and Linda said yes. At one of our sessions she actually broke down and felt like she had moved past something. That helped me better understand how she processed horrible memories and that it was okay to continue our work.

Linda's first marriage had broken apart due to her past. As we continued, she felt as if she would be able to move forward into another relationship. Nervous that she had not had any sexual relations in many years, she thought that any man she may meet would not be patient or understanding of her past abuse. Linda was learning that it was okay to let the past go and to move forward toward her dream of meeting another man and having a healing relationship.

By session twelve Linda made great strides. She was able to go through our last session with no breaks and told me that she felt great! I was elated for her. She asked me why it took so many years to find that type of help. I told her that eventually, once properly educated, medical and holistic professionals could work together one day.

Medicine is medicine, and holism is holism. Some physicians try to integrate into the field of alternative medicine, but many do not succeed. Consumers become so disheartened with medicine that they do not want to see one more medical doctor. Then there are professionals in my field who try to be medical. A definite disconnect has taken place. Practitioners need to choose the training that is most near and dear to their hearts and go with it, without hurting the trusting people they are caring for.

Eventually Linda met a genuinely nice man who gave her the space she needed to continue on her path to healing. They later married. Linda kept in touch for a while. She would send me an e-mail just to thank me for the opportunity to work with me. Her e-mails were always upbeat. It pleases me that I could help her. It took some patience on my part to work slowly and be understanding of her past, but I am so glad that Linda is healing.

~17~ *Polycystic Ovary Syndrome*

"When you get to the end of your rope, tie a knot and hang on."

—Franklin D. Roosevelt

Candace, age twenty-eight, and her husband came to see me because they were having trouble conceiving. Based on the information I had gathered, it sounded like she may have been suffering from polycystic ovary syndrome. In helping me identify the symptoms of possible PCOS, she told me that her periods were almost nonexistent and there were no signs of ovulation.

We had an in-depth discussion regarding normal hormonal trends during the menstrual cycle. As I asked more questions of Candace, she told me that she had not had a "normal" twenty-eight-day cycle since she was twenty-four. This always throws up a red flag in my mind to think further about lifestyle. Come to find out, Candace had finished college at age twenty-four and started working for her family's business. Her working situation was clearly stressful, and her diet consisted of a lot of fast food and diet soda. She worked forty hours a week and had no time to continue with her studies to become a teacher.

I do not diagnose medical conditions; however, Candace fit the exact description of PCOS. Her body was top heavy; her face appeared very round (this is called moon face); she was void of menses; she experienced constant pelvic pressure; her lower back always felt strained; she had a lot of acne on her back, chest, and face; she did not ovulate; and, despite her best attempts at the gym, she could not lose her belly fat. Prior to our appointment, Candace had visited her ob-gyn for her routine yearly exam. Her Pap smear had come back normal and the doctor wanted to start her on Clomid.

Clomid is a drug used when problems with ovulation are apparent. If a woman has irregular cycles or anovulatory cycles, Clomid may be tried as a first line of therapy. Clomid is often used in the treatment of PCOS-related infertility. It may also be used in cases of unexplained infertility or when a couple prefers not to use more expensive and invasive fertility treatments like IVF. Clomid may also be used during an IUI procedure.

Clomid's side effects aren't bad, as far as fertility drugs are concerned. The most common side effects are hot flashes, breast tenderness, mood swings, and nausea. But once the medication is stopped, the side effects leave too. The side effect most people are familiar with is the risk of multiples. Women taking Clomid have a 10 percent chance of having twins, but triplets or multiples of more are rare, happening less than 1 percent of the time.

One of the more annoying side effects is the possible decrease in quality of cervical mucus (which sperm needs to make their way to the egg), making conception more difficult. Clomid can also make the lining of the uterus thinner and less ideal for implantation. This is why more is not necessarily better when it comes to Clomid dosage and use.

Clomid jumpstarts ovulation in 80 percent of patients, and 40–45 percent of women using Clomid will get pregnant within six cycles of use. Using Clomid for more than six cycles is not generally recommended. If six cycles go by and pregnancy is not achieved, other alternatives may be considered.

Any woman starting a stimulation drug like Clomid should be given a pelvic ultrasound. Usually a physician will want to examine the condition of the ovaries and make a plan from there. PCOS ovaries have a typical pattern. Called "string of pearls," the pattern emerges as the cysts on the ovarian surface line up next to each other, resembling a row of pearls. Success rates for induction of ovulation vary considerably and depend on the age of the woman, type of medication used, and whether other factors are presenting in the couple.

Candace felt that Clomid would not be a good fit for her.

After gathering her history, I had some great ideas on how to approach her situation. We did a full saliva hormone panel and noted very elevated testosterone and DHEA levels, which is another characteristic of PCOS. I started her on an herbal and vitamin regimen to help combat her symptoms. We spoke about dietary changes and relaxation methods and started Merciér Therapy. We did our work together over a period of one month. Our sessions would last thirty to forty-five minutes each time. Sometimes the sessions would produce some discomfort, but mostly they were pleasurable and comforting. After just six sessions Candace noticed a crampy feeling in her pelvis. For the first time in many months she was experiencing a menses. We both were excited.

While finishing up our last few sessions together, Candace told me that she felt taller and could take deeper breaths, like she was more open. I always like to hear of such positive feelings. Our work was not finished though. I continued to monitor her cycles and gave her advice on when to start testing for ovulation. It turned out that she did not ovulate for the next three cycles but did continue with a regular menstruation. By the fourth cycle she was noticing ovulatory signs: fertile cervical mucus on cycle days twelve through fifteen and an LH surge on cycle day sixteen. No pregnancy resulted from that cycle. However, by her eighth ovulatory cycle she became pregnant.

Candace ultimately miscarried at twelve weeks, and a doctor discovered that the pregnancy was a blighted ovum. I suggested that she see a reproductive endocrinologist. After starting a workup with the RE, Candace told me that her ovaries appeared cystic and that it was suggested that she start taking the prescribed drug regimen for PCOS. Candace tried to conceive for four cycles using Clomid and HCG trigger injections along with IUI. Her ovaries did not fare well with that protocol. Once determined that she would need a stronger stimulation, she started a regimen of Follistim and HCG trigger. Follitropin beta (Follistim) is a hormone identical to follicle-stimulating hormone produced by the pituitary gland. FSH helps to develop eggs in the ovaries.

Eating a nutritious diet of all organic foods and drinking plenty of water are key. Women with PCOS are at a high risk of insulin resistance and diabetes. That glucose-to-insulin ratio is of utmost importance. Checking the thyroid is also important. If the thyroid is out of balance, then that is good enough birth control for your body.

Candace is pregnant again and is hopeful for the future. I know that if Candace continued following my holistic protocol and the RE's regimen, she would have a much more solid chance of being successful. It is not one or the other. Both approaches work together in symphony, and it requires a commitment on your part. I have helped several women with PCOS become pregnant. I can honestly tell you that is not an easy road, but it can be accomplished.

~18~ Teenage Girls with
Menstrual Dysfunction and Pelvic Pain

"If the pain wanders, do not waste your time with doctors."

—Mignon McLaughlin

More and more I receive calls from mothers of teenage girls with moderate to intense menstrual pain. A typical dialogue sounds something like this: "My daughter has been experiencing painful periods for several months and we went to our family doctor for help. Dr. Smith has recommended that Debbie start taking a birth control pill to help with her discomfort. Both Debbie and I agree that this would not be a good decision for her. We really would like to know how to approach this from a more natural standpoint."

Fifteen-year-old Debbie and her mom came in to discuss Merciér Therapy and a gentle herbal regimen to help combat the problem. Upon our first visit I took a medical and gynecological history. I suggested that we start using pelvic therapy right away. It was important for Debbie to make the commitment to herself and stick to a regimen of therapeutic work. Her uterus needed repositioning, and the surrounding structures had become tight with trigger points. Next we talked about diet and exercise. I impressed upon Debbie the importance of eating only organic foods. Once our six-week pelvic therapy regimen was finished, Debbie was able to move more freely and felt more movement within her hips and lower back. The pain from her menses was gone due to a physical therapeutic massage modality. No drugs used and no unwanted side effects noted.

Many times I find that these young ladies are eating a poor diet lacking in protein. Protein forms an important nutrient component of the body. Made up of essential and nonessential amino acids, it helps in building and repairing muscles and bones, restoring body cells, providing a source of energy, and controlling many of the important metabolism processes in the body.

Our bodies get protein from the food we eat. Unarguably, protein derived from animals, in the form of meat and milk, has the highest concentration of protein, because it contains all nine essential amino acids. Vegetable protein, on the other hand, lacks one or more essential amino acids, which is why it is considered incomplete.

Vegans and vegetarians need to consume a wide variety of protein-rich vegetables so they can get all their essential amino acids. Depending on weight, an average protein intake for an adult is 50–70 grams per day. Review the list in the back of this book to gain a better idea of what and how much needs to be consumed daily.

Protein deficiency symptoms:

- Edema—a collection of fluid under the skin, most commonly affecting the legs, feet, and ankles, but can occur anywhere on the body
- Weight loss
- Thinning or brittle hair, hair loss
- Ridges or deep lines in fingernails and toenails
- Skin becomes very light, burns easily in the sun
- Reduced pigmentation in the hair on scalp and body
- Skin rashes, dryness, flakiness
- General weakness and lethargy
- Muscle soreness and weakness, cramps

- ○ Menstrual irregularities and pain

- ○ Slowness in healing wounds, cuts, scrapes, and bruises

- ○ Bedsores and other skin ulcers

- ○ Difficulty sleeping

- ○ Headache

- ○ Nausea and stomach pain

- ○ Fainting

I met with sixteen-year-old Jenny and her mother to discuss her menstrual history. Cycle day one was average, and her bleeding was rather light with no cramping. Cycle day two was the day Jenny needed to stay home from school due to intense back pain and low frontal cramping. In fact, her pain was so bad that she had trouble moving from her bed to the washroom. In prior cycles she had taken an over-the-counter pain reliever. After the fifth cycle of pain, she was finding no relief with the pain medicine. Her mother took her to see a medical doctor, who suggested that Jenny start a birth control pill. This suggestion is par for the allopathic course. Medical doctors know how to prescribe medications and often do not think any credible holistic resources are available. Luckily Jenny's mother was thinking outside the narrow resources of her medical doctor and made an appointment to consult with me.

Jenny was an athlete and had taken a fall on her tailbone a year earlier. I asked her if she noticed if the pain started after the fall. She really had to think about it, yet in fact after the fall was when she noticed her periods getting intense. Next I asked Jenny if she had any blood clotting during her menstrual cycle. She told me that she did notice some clots but only on cycle days two and three, when her pain was the most intense. Suspecting a uterine malposition, I asked Jen to empty her bladder so I could palpate around her lower abdomen. I found that her uterus was anteverted and pulled off to the right. The uterus was literally stuck in the ilium. The nearby psoas and iliacus (hip flexors) were also involved and very tight. Many trigger points were found within the right hip and sacroiliac joint, the joint between the tail bone and pelvic bone. All structures on the left had been greatly lengthened to accommodate the contracted tissue on the right. I then knew a great deal of work needed to be done.

Jenny's first session was the first day of her period, so she feared what kind of pain the next day would bring. As I started my work, she felt only slight discomfort. I asked her to feel her lower abdomen prior to starting the session and once again when we completed the session. Jenny could not believe that everything felt so softened. When she got off my table, she told me she felt taller and could take a nice, deep, expansive breath without any pain at all. We discussed diet. I put her on supportive herbs and scheduled her next appointment.

The next day I received a call from Jenny. She did not know what I had done, she said, but her period had completely gone away and she felt great. Also, she wanted to know why her period was gone. I told her that working with an organ and helping restore blood flow and function is like turning on a light switch. It took four days for her period to return, and once it did Jenny said that her bleeding was a normal flow with virtually no pain. With therapy, there are bound to be some immediate changes and some that are gradual. All in all she was pleased at the end of our sessions and felt great. Jenny's periods are now twenty-eight-day cycles with no more menstrual or lower back pain.

Part 3

Final Words

~19~ *Proper Diet*

"In order to change we must be sick and tired of being sick and tired."

—Author Unkown

When a woman decides to work with a medical practice to help her conceive, so many crucial processes are left by the wayside. Nutrition is one of them. I used to have an office next to a mortgage company. Its receptionist was undergoing her third IVF attempt and I asked how it was going for her. She told me that it was stressful and that she just wanted to be done with the whole thing. (Whenever I'd see her during her cycles, she was always in a terrible mood.) A few days after our conversation, she went in for her embryo transfer. Two of her five embryos had successfully thawed and had been placed back into her uterus. About two weeks later I saw her again and asked how she was doing. The transfer had been unsuccessful, she said, and she had spent over sixty thousand dollars. I was sorry to hear the news and urged her to come see me. Later that day I saw her in our office complex parking lot with a cigarette, cola, and chips. You have got to be kidding me, I thought. Obviously no one had told her that for optimal growth babies do not smoke, drink cola, and eat a poor diet. No one had counseled her to better health while going through IVF. In essence, she and her husband wasted time, money, and emotions.

The American diet consists of many chemically enhanced and processed foods. What will happen if you eat a diet of processed foods? The chemicals will create an inflammatory process in your body, throwing your immune system into a tailspin, as well as making you overweight and irritable. Any time inflammation occurs, the body's natural defense is to create a fibrous, glue-like adhesive on or around your visceral organs. Right now, more than any other time in U.S. history, our nation is facing a huge rise in cases of chronic fatigue syndrome and fibromyalgia. Both diseases stem from inflammation. Big surprise, given the diet we are eating.

A great deal of media coverage centers on improving our nation's food quality. Jamie Oliver, a chef from England, has challenged some of our most unhealthy cities to make dietary changes to include more home-cooked, healthful meals. Author Michael Pollan has written wonderful books to aid our understanding of our nation's food crisis. And a great documentary called *Food, Inc.* will assist you in making better decisions when meal planning.

In general, it's best to avoid the following ingredients:

- Sodium nitrite
- Saccharin, aspartame, acesulfame-K
- Caffeine
- Olestra
- Artificial coloring

In addition to suggesting a diet of organic fruits, vegetables, nuts, seeds, whole grains, eggs, and dairy, I use a specific protocol of herbs and vitamins to create natural wellness and enhance women's chances of conception.

Your diet during pregnancy needs your utmost attention. During pregnancy and lactation, your need for protein significantly increases. For the duration of pregnancy, experts recommend that protein intake be a minimum of sixty grams per day. Women carrying twins or another multiple pregnancy need even more. Protein is required for the physical growth and cellular development of your baby. It is also required for the placenta, amniotic tissues, and maternal tissues. Further, your blood volume increases by 50 percent during pregnancy, and protein is needed to produce new blood cells and circulating proteins. Animal proteins should be eaten minimally unless they are grass fed and organically sourced. Carefully consider your purchase of commercially farmed animals for human consumption, since they are fed hormones, steroids, and antibiotics. Our bodies do not need bovine and porcine antibiotics.

Empower yourself and become educated about food. Let it be your medicine. I am not a fan of loading up on supplements. Why take so many supplements if you could get those nutrients from your food? Convenience is why people take pills rather than just eating the foods. Simply put. After all, we are a country of convenience.

Keeping your diet simple can be uncomplicated. Eat real foods. Stop buying no-fat, low-fat, low-calorie, no calorie. Eat butter and plant fats like avocado. Eat nuts like almonds and walnuts. Eat plenty of bright-colored foods. Every day I sit down and eat a huge, bright-colored salad and feel really good after I have eaten it! My salad bowl looks something like this: organic spinach, bell pepper, pomegranate seeds, avocado, blueberries, walnuts, dried cranberries, beets, broccoli, and cheese topped with red wine vinegar and olive oil. Yummy and so fulfilling. Your bowels will be happier, and so will you. Eating clean foods will keep your inflammatory response at a minimum and your risk of scar tissue formation low.

So much more helpful information is available in the nutrition arena. You can find resources, including a list of proteins, in the back of this book. I encourage you to buy organic foods whenever possible. Organic fruits, vegetables, grains, and dairy will help keep nutrients flowing and bowel movements regular and healthy. And make sure you take a solid prenatal vitamin. I recommend Maternal Symmetry from Vitanica.

Then after you deliver, I encourage you to encapsulate your placenta. Ingesting the placenta as a dried supplement has many benefits. Visit www.placentabenefits.info to read of its advantages.

Nutrition is key to a healthy body. I will come halfway and help, but you have to commit to come the other half. Never expect anyone to do the work for you. Do it yourself and reap the grand rewards of great pelvic health.

~20~ Tips for Healing on Your Own

"The best six doctors anywhere,
And no one can deny it,
Are sunshine, water, rest, and air,
Exercise and diet.
These six will gladly you attend,
If only you are willing.
Your mind they'll ease,
Your will they'll mend,
And charge you not one shilling."

—Nursery rhyme quoted by Wayne Fields
in *What the River Knows*

I wholeheartedly believe that our bodies have the ability to fully recover from many physical pains. With your commitment, only you have the ability to make changes in your daily routine. The first item—and perhaps the most difficult—is changing your diet to facilitate the healing that you so need. Second is incorporating movement. Think about your body, or, for that matter, anything that breathes. A living, breathing thing cannot live optimally without movement. It just makes sense.

After my pelvic laparoscopies, I turned to Pilates to help me regain movement with my general rehabilitation. Remember, I had three pelvic surgeries to clean up very aggressive stage four endometriosis. After each surgery, scar tissue had built up and could have caused major organ dysfunction, trigger points, and muscular restriction. Let me help you understand Pilates.

Pilates is a physical fitness system developed in the early twentieth century by Joseph Pilates in Germany. He believed his method used the mind to control the muscles. The Pilates program focuses on core postural muscles, which help keep the body balanced and are essential to providing support for the spine. The pelvis muscles are referred to as the core. They form an internal muscular corset that works together to stabilize the spine and pelvis. Visualize this as a box: the abdominals in the front, the spinal muscles in the back, the diaphragm as the ceiling, and the pelvic floor as the bottom.

In essence, the pelvic floor is strong but can become weakened by events such as childbirth, obesity, and menopause, when estrogen levels drop. A weakened pelvic floor can contribute to incontinence initially and may even cause a genital prolapse. First signs of a weakened pelvic floor are little leaks of urine when coughing, sneezing, or running.

Hormones of pregnancy also affect the pelvis. During pregnancy, hormonal changes alter the stiffness of the ligaments, making them more lax. This allows the body to prepare for the birthing process by permitting greater mobility. However, this means that the muscles of the pelvis become even more important in stabilizing the spine and the pelvis. If pelvic muscles are weak, a woman may develop lower back pain.

Pilates exercises teach awareness of breathing and alignment of the spine and aim to strengthen the deep muscles of the pelvis and torso.

Many fitness centers offer Pilates classes and often will incorporate their own twists on the movements. Mat classes are great, but you really need to try using the Cadillac and the reformer. Both of these pieces of equipment have helped me learn better form. Correct form and breathing are deeply important, and that is why I highly encourage you to find a trained instructor at a Pilates studio. In my search I found an excellent teacher by the name of Serena Smith at Fox River Pilates Center in Geneva, Illinois. Serena's education and background in dance have helped her to even better understand that movement is a crucial part of our lives. We worked together during thirty-five private sessions. For many years prior to finding Pilates, I had worked out in a gym with a trainer. Never had I found such deep gratification with any other training than I had with Pilates. My body actually started to wake up and be able to move in ways that it had not moved in a long time. Pilates helped me feel longer, stronger, and leaner. After six sessions I already knew that a change had occurred. I love Pilates so much that I bought a reformer and chair so I could continue my training at home. Thank you, Serena. You are an awesome teacher!

Next I would like you to explore using the foam roller. With the foam roller you'll be able to release fascial restrictions in your back and pelvis. I recommend the Smartroller by OPTP. In my opinion this roller is by far superior to others out there. Buy a guide as well to learn how to use the Smartroller. Go slowly, and use it every day. As you work, you'll notice areas of restriction and discomfort. Work only as much as your body allows. If you push yourself too much, you may injure yourself.

The next part of your journey to healing your pelvis is vaginal steam treatments, which can be done at home in complete privacy. Let me tell you that everything I talk about I have tried myself. I am a proactive partner concerning my health and will do my best to avoid unnecessary medical interventions. I have been using vaginal steam treatments in my own healing for many years. They have been used in Europe for centuries and have proven healthy results. Here's how to get started.

Vaginal Steam Treatment

1. Purchase a small slow cooker that has a low heat setting. Place the pouch of Merciér Therapy herbs into the pot of hot water. Let the packet steep for three minutes.

2. Place a chair that resembles a toilet over the pot. I recommend a birthing stool with legs so you are not too close to the heat. The goal here is to not burn yourself.

3. Undress from your waist down, and make sure you have a large towel to wrap around your waist.

4. Place a small towel on the area where you will be sitting. It should be soft and comfy on your sitz (ischium) bones.

5. Sit on the birthing stool, letting your lower back and hips relax as the steam heads upward onto the pelvic floor. Your vagina will start to feel more open and supple.

6. Stay in this position on the birthing stool for fifteen or so minutes. If the heat becomes too hot, then adjust the temperature of the slow cooker. The heat should never feel uncomfortable.

7. Once you have finished, make time to just relax.

Vaginal steam is healthy for releasing the tight areas of musculature within the pelvic floor. Once those muscles are relaxed, then typically the ligaments within the whole pelvis become more flexible. I would recommend that you steam at least once per month for general relaxation and once or twice per week in times of pain. Follow the steam treatment with twenty or so Kegal exercises.

Next I want to talk about whole body movement. Speaking of release and flexibility, I find that dancing is liberating and lubricating. Deliberate movement of your body will lubricate your joints and help awaken your proprioceptors—those cells within the muscle tissue that enable important sensory movements. When the cells become activated, you may also gain new levels of flexibility. As women, we need that extra movement within our pelvis anyway.

Our pelvis holds a very dear organ that is deeply connected to our heart; that organ is our womb.

Another valuable practice is focused breathing in a meditative or quiet state. Here's how to start: Find a comfy, quiet place to lie down. Place your hands on your belly and take a deep breath. If you find that your chest has risen on your inhale, then you have just taken a paradoxical breath. Paradoxical means the opposition between the diaphragm muscle and the abdominal muscles. You have just forced air into your lungs and negated to bring air deep into your abdomen. Now try this: Take another breath, but this time inhale and make your belly rise. Count silently to four on the inhale and hold when your belly is extended to its fullest. Now release that breath to the count of four. Enjoy this for about fifteen minutes and then go about your day.

It's far more effective to meditate every day at the same time for fifteen minutes than randomly once a week for an hour. A busy schedule does make it tricky to find the opportunity to consistently meditate, so select a time that works best for you. Try meditating in the morning upon waking and before getting out of bed, or maybe in the evening or after work would be better. Only you know your schedule and its demands. Meditating will help you get centered during your day. Complication abounds in our lives. Do make a time commitment to yourself. Keep your appointment with yourself.

Music can also play a part in healing. Some of my favorite music comes from Karen Drucker. Karen's music is inspiring, creative, and playful and has brought me a lot of joy. Sometimes I like to listen to her softer tunes for a more meditative effect, and then there are those more powerful songs that I listen to loudly! The words in Karen's music have taught me so much over the years, and I have learned to appreciate myself more from just listening to her lyrics. Listen for yourself and then get up and dance, dance, dance! Remember, movement is key for good overall pelvic health.

Next, are you looking around at a cluttered home or workspace? If you are, ask yourself why those spaces are messy. Any kind of clutter creates an obstacle to the smooth flow of energy around a space.

This in turn creates "stuckness" and confusion in our lives: it blocks our creativity, it prevents us from moving forward, it hinders our relationships, and it provides an environment that doesn't support us. When coming home after a long day, you want to sit and relax. Are you really able to relax knowing that your space is in disarray? Like it or not, we are all products of our surroundings. I keep my house as tidy and organized as possible. This way I know where everything is and do not frustrate myself when looking for something. A tidy workspace, too, is important to me and of equal importance to the women who see me for care. If my office were untidy, I am sure I would not be a grounded practitioner and may not be able to complete my work as efficiently as I do now. Clutter will clog up your mind. Declutter, and enjoy your newfound inner peace.

My home and office are places of peace. Sometimes I spray essential oils to open up that space and clear out old energies. The essential oils of peace and energy are there for your use. The best essential oils are pure with no artificial chemicals. Young Living Essential Oils are some of the finest. Blends called Joy, Awaken, Inspiration, Inner Child, and Gentle Baby are all my personal favorites. The amazing names alone hint of how wonderful the oils smell. To make a simple room spray, use spring water and ten or so drops of your favorite oils. You can buy a glass bottle with a spray top and simply spritz right into the air to create a lovely smelling environment. You'll be surprised at the feelings that may arise upon spraying something that will aid you in your process of wellness, but also note that this is something you created. Aromatherapy is a great form of self-reliant healing. While it is not a miracle cure, it may help ease pain, promote faster healing, and uplift your spirits.

Burning candles is another way to bring a soft, compassionate light to any environment. I especially like to light them when doing pelvic therapy. Some of my clients using IVF drugs have become sensitive to smells, so scented candles are not necessary. A softly lit room is peaceful and reflects a certain mood. If you are able to tolerate the scent of an essential oil, then light a stress-releasing aromatherapy candle (lavender, chamomile, patchouli, geranium, or rose), take a few deep breaths, and allow your mind to clear.

A clean environment helps us think clearer, make better decisions, and live a more comforting life.

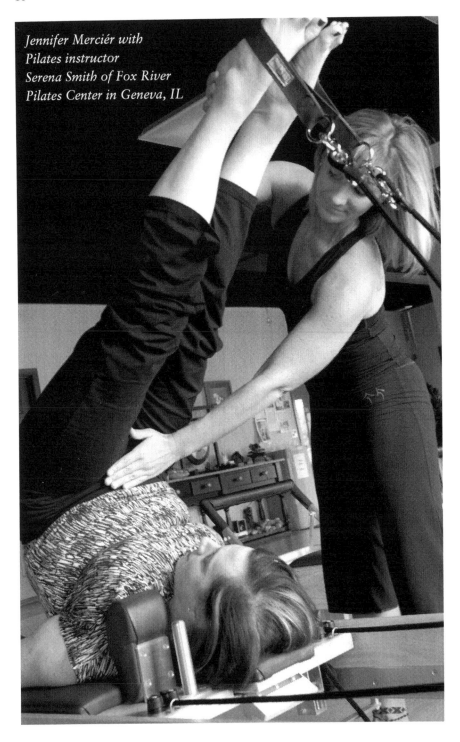

Jennifer Merciér with Pilates instructor Serena Smith of Fox River Pilates Center in Geneva, IL

~21~ Avoiding Birth Trauma

"Adopt the pace of nature: her secret is patience."

—Ralph Waldo Emerson

In my years of practice I have received many phone calls from pregnant women who were feeling uncomfortable with their obstetricians' decision to force labor. "My OB wants to induce my labor at thirty-nine weeks because my baby is too big." "My OB is going out of town and wants to make sure I deliver while he is still in the office." "If I don't go into labor by forty weeks, then my OB is planning to induce." "If I don't progress within a certain amount of time after induction, then I'll need a C-section." I may have heard every excuse to start a woman's labor, and unless those excuses involve sincere medical risk factors, they are nonsense. There is no need to force a baby out when he or she is not ready. It is amazing, but babies come when they are good and ready. The process is not one that is broken and in need of a mechanical and intervening delivery.

In terms of forced labor and delivery regarding the muscles and organs of the pelvis, we should be trying to preserve the natural integrity of the pelvic floor. Multiple births have a strong association of weakening the visceral organs as well as the pelvic organs.

As an experienced practitioner, I have realized that it is not the number of childbirths that is important but rather the manner in which the births are carried out. Women who deliver with forceps or suction, whereby the child is "pulled out" without regard to contractions, have their perineum drawn downward at the moment when the tissues, under the influence of hormones, are relaxed and very stretchable. If the obstetrician has a slightly heavy hand, some of the tissues will never regain their original position and elasticity. Add to this an episiotomy and the associated scar tissue, and you will find all of the necessary conditions for a variety of abdominopelvic dysfunctions. Suction should be considered only in cases of labor dystocia and is certainly not indispensable. It can have a multitude of adverse effects on the newborn as well as the mother. Wishing to force the body is an allopathic concept. The more holistic approach is to restore natural function by giving a gentle nudge.

In my midwifery training I experienced hospital, birth center, and home births. By far, a home birth has proven time and time again to be the most safe, personal, and warm experience for both mother and baby. I have seen women in hospitals be literally run over by medical staff taking over the process and experience. A woman giving birth in a hospital becomes disconnected, and the birth becomes a medical procedure. Please know that I am not discouraging you from having your baby in a hospital. I am, rather, sharing with you years of experience.

Giving birth is not a medical event, but in the United States this is what it has become. Stay connected to your pregnancy by educating yourself. Women today have many options for labor support and preparatory education classes. Too many times, though, these great resources are not utilized or just not recommended. Many pregnant women start care with an obstetrician, a trained surgeon. The pregnancy then becomes a diagnosis, and the prenatal care involves not educating but rather managing the birth using "proven" medical protocols and influencing the woman into feeling that her body is inadequate to birth the baby the way women have for so many years. Not all obstetricians intend to manipulate women away from staying connected to their pregnancy, but this is true in 80 percent of the cases I have observed. Practitioners need to allow women to do the work that their bodies are quite capable of handling. One of our greatest mistakes as women is to hand ourselves entirely over to another person to manipulate. For someone to take control of us is an assault on our intelligence.

How would you go about planning for an important event in your life? You would take careful measure to ensure the safety, enjoyment, and comfort of yourself, your partner, family, and friends. You would not let your wedding planner take over all of your visions for a great wedding event without creative input from you. You would not let your travel agent plan your entire vacation, ignoring your ideas for seeing certain attractions. You see where I'm going with these examples. Trained professionals are available to assist you with choosing certain options—options you've shown interest in—and now your wishes are being respected.

You may choose to have a relatively noninvasive hospital birth if you voice your needs and stay firm. However, your medical provider has to respect your choices. Collaborate with your physician. Each step of the way you need to be included in your care. What is important to you? How do you envision your labor? Have you even thought about it? Ultimately I would recommend that you have a doula present during your labor and birth. A doula will greatly increase your chances of upholding your wishes for a nonmedical birth.

By the way, listen to only favorable stories about pregnancy, labor, and birth. Most women give away their birthing experience to the medical profession, leaving them with nothing but negative stories. Negative stories are told from a fearful angle and have no benefit to you. Positive stories, on the other hand, will help you have a beautiful birth.

Take charge of your pregnancy so you feel confident with your choices. Happy birthing!

Thank You, God, for making this book possible. I will envision its circulation into the hands of women and practitioners who need the information to help themselves and their patients. It is Your grace and love that have compelled me to write this book.

Resources

Choosing to Eat Well

- *Jonny Bowden, The 150 Healthiest Foods on Earth* (Beverly, MA: Fair Winds Press, 2007).

- Michael Pollan, *Food Rules: An Eater's Manual* (New York, NY: Penguin Group USA Inc., 2009).

- *Food, Inc.*, DVD, directed by Robert Kenner (New York, NY: Magnolia Pictures, 2008).

- *Food Matters*, DVD, directed by James Colquhoun and Laurentine ten Bosch (Metuchen, NJ: Passion River Films, 2009).

- *The Future of Food*, DVD, directed by Deborah Koons Garcia (New York, NY: Virgil Films and Entertainment, 2005).

- *Killer at Large*, DVD, directed by Steven Greenstreet (New York, NY: The Disinformation Company, 2009).

- *Processed People: The Documentary*, DVD, directed by Jeff Nelson (Porter Ranch, CA: Mostly Magic Productions, 2009).

- Weston A. Price Foundation (www.westonaprice.org). Good information about food, farming, and healing.

Protein List

- Eggs (1 medium size) 6 g
- Egg white, dried (100g) 79–95 g
- Milk (1 glass) 19 g
- Soya milk, plain (200 ml) 6 g
- Tofu (100 g) 8 g
- Low-fat yogurt, plain (150g) 8 g
- Cod fillets (100g, or 3.5 ounces) 21 g
- Whitefish, smoked, dried (100g) 67 g
- Salmon (100g) 39.9 g
- Cheddar cheese (100g, or 3.5 ounces) 25 g
- Parmesan cheese, grated (100g) 38.5 g
- Roast beef (100g, or 3.5 ounces) 28 g
- Roast chicken (100g, or 3.5 ounces) 25 g
- Other meats (100g, or 3.5 ounces) 25 g
- Sausages (100g, or 3.5 ounces) 12 g
- Bacon (100g, or 3.5 ounces) 25 g
- Pork, cured, bacon, cooked, pan-fried (100g) 38.3 g
- Ham (100g, or 3.5 ounces) 18 g
- Beef burgers, freezer type (100g) 20 g
- Corned beef (100g, or 3.5 ounces) 26 g
- Luncheon meat (100g, or 3.5 ounces) 13 g
- Soy protein isolate (100g) 80 g
- Whey protein isolate (100g) 79.5 g
- Soybeans, dry, roasted (100g) 39.6 g
- Peanut butter (15ml) 7 g
- Broccoli (80 grams) 2 g

- Almonds (1/4 cup) 8 g
- Peanuts (1/4 cup) 9 g
- Cashews (1/4 cup) 5 g

Supplements

Vitanica has a wonderful product line. I carry almost all of their products in my office. If you are a licensed practitioner, call Doug or Estelle and ask for a product catalog. Vitanica also has a consumer line that is carried at many health food stores and online (www.vitanica.com).

Traditional Osteopathy

- The Barral Institute (www.barralinstitute.com).
- Canadian College of Osteopathy (www.osteopathiecollege.com).

Pregnancy-Related Resources

- Belly Bandit (www.bellybandit.com). The supportive band helps support your uterus postbirth. Every woman needs one!
- The Sacro Wedgy is awesome for helping to correct the balance within the pelvic bones (www.sacrowedgy.com).
- The Birth Trauma Association (www.birthtraumaassociation.org.uk).
- Placenta encapsulation (www.placentabenefits.info).
- *The Business of Being Born*, DVD, directed by Abby Epstein (New York, NY: New Line Cinema, 2007).

Music for Healing

- *o*   Karen Drucker's music is empowering and creative (www.karendrucker.com).

- *o*   Plumb is a Christian artist whose voice is very serene. I recommend the Blink CD (www.plumbinfo.com).

Aromatherapy

Young Living Essential Oils has some of the finest essential oil blends. I use them in practice and just love them (www.youngliving.com).

Tools for Fitness

- *o*   Serena Smith and Ben Basar own Fox River Pilates Center in Geneva, Illinois (www.foxriverpilates.com). They are wonderful!

- *o*   With the Smartroller from OPTP you'll be able to release fascial restrictions in your back and pelvis (www.optp.com/ SMARTROLLER_SMR36.aspx).

Glossary

abdominal viscera—The organs in the abdominal cavity: stomach, intestines, liver, spleen, pancreas, and parts of the urinary and reproductive tracts.

allopathic doctor—A doctor of western medicine.

autoimmune diseases—Diseases in which the body fights its own natural processes.

blighted ovum—An oocyte (egg) that contains no genetic material.

embryo—Meaning "that which grows," "embryo" describes a human in the early stage of fetal growth, from conception to the first eight weeks of pregnancy.

embryo transfer—A procedure done after eggs have been retrieved and fertilized, resulting in an embryo. The embryo is then transferred into the uterus.

embryologist—A doctor specializing in embryo development from its fertilization to the fetus stage.

endometrial biopsy—A small amount of endometrium (uterine lining) is removed during an office procedure to evaluate the endometrial cells for abnormalities.

endometriomas—Blood-filled cystic masses that form on the ovaries, typically when a woman has endometriosis.

endometriosis—A retrograde, or backing up, of endometrial cells out of the fallopian tubes into the lower pelvic cavity and abdomen. The endometrial cells start to adhere to the surrounding organs—such as the bladder, small intestine, rectum, ovaries, and uterus—and bleed during a normal menstrual period, causing pain and adhesions.

endometrium—Uterine lining.

fascia—Connective tissue.

follicle-stimulating hormone (FSH)—A hormone released that helps fertility specialists determine how many eggs a woman has in reserve.

human chorionic gonadotropin (HCG)—A hormone released during pregnancy.

in vitro fertilization (IVF)—An ooctye (egg) and sperm are placed together in a lab to make an embryo.

intrauterine insemination (IUI)—Sperm are injected with a tiny catheter directly into a woman's uterus.

Kegal exercises—A type of pelvic floor exercise. Contract your pelvic floor muscles, the muscles you would use to stop urinating (without flexing the muscles in your abdomen, thighs, or buttocks). Hold the contraction for five to ten seconds, then relax for five to ten seconds. Repeat ten times three times a day.

laparoscopy—An operation in the abdomen or pelvis involving the aid of a camera through small incisions. It is intended to either diagnose or repair a condition.

luteal phase—The time in a woman's cycle after ovulation.

menarche—The first menstrual period.

naprapath—A doctor who performs a modality of various soft tissue manipulations.

oocyte—Female zygote (egg).

overstimulation—This can happen when a woman undergoing assisted reproductive procedures such as IVF or IUI is given too much follicular stimulating drug. The ovaries become very full with too many follicles (egg sacs).

ovum—Female egg.

pathology—A diagnosis that is not normal.

reproductive endocrinologist (RE)—A doctor specializing in treating people with reproductive disorders.

stimulation cycle—Beginning part of a medically assisted cycle like IVF or IUI.

tenaculum—An instrument used to hold the cervix and keep the uterus in place during gynecological procedures.

thyroid—A gland that regulates the metabolism.

trigger points—Hardened or tight area within the muscular tissue, causing pain.

xiphoid process—The area between the ribs at the lower end of the sternum (breast bone).

Index

Professionals interested in taking a Merciér Therapy training class should contact our office at 847-628-9570 or visit www.merciertherapy.com.

Clients interested in undergoing Merciér Therapy are encouraged to contact our office at 847-628-9570 or visit www.drjennifermercier.com.

Clients outside Illinois can complete the Shared Journey Fertility Program within a four-day weekend.